A MOTHER IS BORN

A
MOTHER
IS BORN

Preparing

for

Motherhood

During

Pregnancy

Merete Leonhardt-Lupa

Bergin & Garvey
Westport, Connecticut • London

Library of Congress Cataloging-in-Publication Data

Leonhardt-Lupa, Merete.
    A mother is born : preparing for motherhood during pregnancy /
Merete Leonhardt-Lupa.
        p. cm.
    Includes bibliographical references and index.
    ISBN 0–89789–353–0 (pbk. : alk. paper)
    1. Motherhood. 2. Pregnancy. I. Title.
HQ759.L468   1995
306.874'3—dc20   94–29716

British Library Cataloguing in Publication Data is available.

Library of Congress Catalog Card Number: 94–29716
ISBN: 0–89789–353–0

First published in 1995

Bergin & Garvey, 88 Post Road West, Westport, CT 06881
An imprint of Greenwood Publishing Group, Inc.

Printed in the United States of America

The paper used in this book complies with the
Permanent Paper Standard issued by the National
Information Standards Organization (Z39.48–1984).

10 9 8 7 6 5 4 3 2 1

CONTENTS

PREFACE

To the reader:

   With this book I wish to offer you help to get a good start in motherhood. I want to show how you in pregnancy can prepare for the mothering experience so that you can meet your child with an open heart. I hope that by encouraging you to examine, clarify, and make use of what is happening to you, I can inspire you to find the essence of your own experience.

   Since I believe the best time to examine the identity changes that takes place when a woman becomes a mother is in the introspective state of pregnancy, I write with the pregnant woman in mind. You do not have to be pregnant to read this book, however. You may already be a mother who is struggling with the mothering role, or you may be contemplating having a child and wonder what motherhood entails. Perhaps you are simply curious about a modern perspective on motherhood. What I have to say is meant to be useful for anyone who needs a deeper understanding of the psychological realities of motherhood.

   When I was pregnant with my first child, I did not know what to expect from motherhood. Excitedly, I grasped for every opportunity to find answers to my concerns and questions. I attended classes on childbirth, breast-feeding, and infant care. I read many books on the same subjects and bombarded every mother in sight with my questions. As the due date came close, I felt well prepared for motherhood.

   One day the stork arrived at my door and to my great surprise he brought my baby boy *and* an unfamiliar woman who was supposed to be the new me. I was bewildered. How could I have been so mindless as to forget that becoming a mother was also about myself? Why had nobody warned me? Now it was too late. Here I was, and I had no idea of who I was, who I was becoming, and how I was going to deal with the changes.

   The demands of my tiny, sweet, and helpless baby boy left me with little time and energy to think about motherhood. My days were filled with feedings, diaper changes, and naps. When I had a few spare moments for reflection I could only think about my poor son, who was suffering from my clumsiness and bad attitude. I painfully had to realize that the preparations I had made in pregnancy had taught me what to expect from the daily care of my baby, but they had not prepared me for the changes I would encounter in myself.

From the interviews I have made since I decided to write about the process of becoming a mother, I know that I am not the only mother who wishes she had prepared herself better for the mothering experience. Unfortunately, many women enter motherhood feeling overwhelmed, frightened and alone with their self-doubts. In pregnancy we typically learn lots of practical skills to handle the demands of childbirth and infant care, but rarely do we get help with the psychological and emotional pain of becoming mothers.

Although I gave birth in the United States, I grew up in the archipelago of the Swedish west coast. Bohuslan is a dramatic meetingplace for the elements of nature. Rocks of ash-gray granite stone rise toward the sky while their sheer walls drop vertically into the water. Salt water from the Atlantic Ocean surrounds the many islands in the area and adds softness and movement to the harsh and barren rocks. Lush trees and wildflower meadows abound despite the harsh weather and meager soil.

The fierce and dramatic landscape of Bohuslan resonates my longing for the same side in my own nature. I am helplessly drawn to the turbulent and tempestuous conditions of my own inner world. I love navigating between the underwater obstacles and experiencing the fear and excitement of not knowing what I will find. Being thrown out to survive under these unsheltered but yielding conditions makes me feel extra alive.

I found this state of mind in pregnancy. My emotional instability both scared and fascinated me. I found it easy to shed my composed and well-behaved front and become as surprising and unpredictable as I desired. I am no longer pregnant, and I am happy that I am not. I have three wonderful boys to keep me busy. Yet, I continue to be fascinated by the wild nature expressed in pregnancy, which I think of as essentially feminine. I believe that in pregnancy we have an exciting opportunity to integrate this ignored side into our female identities. By being open to psychological transformation we give carnal birth to our babies and spiritual birth to ourselves.

Throughout the book I ardently and relentlessly encourage you to explore your own depths. I have little patience with explaining the theories of women's psychological development, nor with analyzing the social and political situation of mothers. I acknowledge their importance for understanding the mothering role, but I prefer to focus on what women can do to bring out their own mothering potential. In my view, paying attention to your inner thoughts and feelings, no matter how irrational they may seem at first, is the best way to prepare for motherhood.

This book is intended to be a guide into the realm of the inner world where the transformation to mother takes place. The first two chapters discuss the preparations women commonly make during their first pregnancy. "Project Baby" explains our tendency to rationalize the preparations in pregnancy at the expense of an emotional and intuitive understanding of what is happening. "The Perfect Mother" analyzes the impossible expectations women often have for motherhood and how these can undermine their best intentions. The third chapter, "A Woman's Way of Mothering," examines the many changes women face *as women* during the transformation. The following three chapters are intended to inspire the reader to find her own strengths as a mother. "Mother Care" gives examples of what a woman can do to nurture herself in pregnancy and motherhood. "A Mother's Body" and "A Mother's Sexuality" show how the female body and sexuality can be sources of strength in mothering. Chapter 8, "Mother Alone, Parent Together," discusses the differences in the female and male transformations. The final chapter, serving as a summation of the book, uses birth as a metaphor for the emergence of the wise mother-self. The book ends at the place where it all really begins: the first meeting with the baby.

Parallel with the didactic text of my book runs the story of a woman's experiences in pregnancy, which illustrates the themes I discuss. These fictive vignettes are also a way of helping you experience some of the emotions that accompany different aspects of pregnancy. A woman's irrational thoughts and behaviors, her emotional reactions, her attitude to the changing body, and her intuitive, creative and sexual powers are vital ingredients in the process of becoming a mother. By weaving these experiences into the informative text, I wish to touch you in a way that allows your own reflections and reactions to motherhood to come to life.

ACKNOWLEDGMENTS

My thanks go to my friends and family, who like good midwives, helped nurture this book to life:

Catharina and Kent for their encouragement during the time of the first obscure conception of my ideas.

My friends Sonja and Kim, whose mothering skills inspired me.

Michelle, to whose loving care I entrusted my two boys when I closed the door to my writing den behind me.

Lee and Tirzah, who helped me find the place inside where this book could take shape.

Evy, whose advice and support meant so much to me at times when I felt discouraged.

Theresa, who generously donated time and talent to illustrate my work.

Last but not least, to Mark, my husband and most ardent editor, who lived with me through three pregnancies and the making of this book, and who repeatedly has shown his love and belief in me.

A MOTHER
IS BORN

INTRODUCTION

The emergency exit! Anna sighs in relief. She has found a way out. Somehow she lost her way after leaving the clinic. She stumbled deeper and deeper into an unfriendly maze of hallways, staircases, and doors that led nowhere. Panic slowly wrapped cold coils around her. Was this a trap? Somewhere she must have made a mistake.

Anna finds a green oasis of grass to sit down on. Phew. This is too much for her. One minute her heart is pounding in excitement, the next it is pounding in fear. What is going on? She must be dreaming. The lab sheet she clenches in her hand—is it telling the truth? What exactly does the answer scribbled across it mean?

She is not dreaming. After many months on the unmerciful pendulum between hope and disappointment, it is finally happening: She is pregnant.

The moment the realization of pregnancy sinks in is a moment so bewildering it is almost impossible to hold on to. For a short moment the infinity of one's past, present, and future is contained in the dark space of the womb. The pregnant woman who welcomes her new condition feels the same sense of wonder and excitement as the innocent child she once was; the same zest for life; the same faith in the future. A new life is created out of the empty space in her womb, and with the creation of the child she herself will find a new way of being.

Becoming a mother affects your life in ways you cannot even begin to imagine. It is one of the most dramatic and profound personal transformations a woman can ever experience. It will change your way of thinking in areas you believed had nothing to do with mothering. It will change how you view the world. It will change how you relate to other people. It will change how you see your past, present, and future.

Your experiences will take you on a breathtaking journey as intense in joy and euphoria as in pain and confusion. It will take a good deal of determination to stay with the process as well as willingness to examine the many conflicting thoughts and emotions you inevitably will encounter. Some women may intuitively have a sense of direction, but most of us will be confused by the depth of this experience and will need guidance so as not to get lost.

The ultimate challenge for you as a mother-to-be is to manage the tension of the unknown and to take the nine months of pregnancy to discover in mind and in heart what becoming a mother entails. This is most likely to happen when you are free to follow your inclinations and allow yourself to be distracted and delighted by the novelty of pregnancy. You must let yourself be carried away by your imagination and be as innocent and full of wonder as you can possibly be. By being radiantly pregnant, a reverence for the creation of life is fostered inside. The impression will support and nourish you as you are transformed.

In this introduction to the journey into motherhood, we will seek to answer some questions about the transformation that takes place when a woman becomes a mother. We will try to understand what makes this time in a woman's life so challenging, why we must actively prepare for motherhood, and what we can do to facilitate the transformation.

Although becoming a mother has always been an ambitious enterprise that requires a woman's willingness to make significant adjustments in her life, our modern society presents us with demands that make motherhood especially challenging today. Compared to previous generations we have many more complex decisions to make about pregnancy, birth, and life with the baby. We are also exposed to many contradictory ideas of what mothers should or should not be doing. All people seem to have an interest in mothers, whether they base their opinions on their professional expertise, or on their political, feminist, religious, or ethnic beliefs.

Considering motherhood is a bit like standing in the cereal aisle of the grocery store. In front of us is an endless row of possibilities, each wrapped in inviting packaging with witty arguments of why we should make this particular cereal the brand of choice. Yet no cereal box can ever impose the same serious consequences for our decisions as motherhood will. The stakes are high and yet there are few foolproof ways to ensure success. We are left on our own to make the best choices for our children and ourselves.

Ideally, the decision to have a child reflects our personal willingness and readiness for the caretaking role. The widespread use of birth control coupled with society's changing attitude toward childlessness has made motherhood a conscious choice. We are in the enviable situation of being able to postpone motherhood and pursue other interests first if we so wish. The freedom of choice is, however, not always easy to bear. A woman may escape the responsibility for the decision by becoming pregnant "by accident" or because her partner wanted a child or because the biological clock told her it had to be now or never.

Once we have made the decision to have a child, we have the opportunity to choose some unconventional ways to parent. We can consider alternatives to the traditional husband and wife team, such as single parenting and lesbian and gay relationships, or we can remain an unmarried couple with children. The possibilities of adopting a child, engaging in surrogate mothering, or being artificially inseminated also challenge our traditional beliefs about motherhood.

Our long list of possibilities continues. In pregnancy, we must decide on what approach to pregnancy and childbirth we prefer our caregivers to have. Nowadays we can influence such important medical decisions as what fetal tests we want to have done, how we want to manage possible complications, and what kind of birthing experience we wish for. We must also look ahead and decide on who will care for the baby after birth. Which parent will stay at home in the beginning? If day care must be arranged, what kind do we prefer and how do we find it?

Once all these decisions are made, we are finally ready to turn to the baby and his or her needs. These arrangements include everything from the practical matters of choosing what baby items to acquire to the mind-boggling question of how to raise the child.

The freedom of choice is in many ways liberating and empowering for women. We can set up a situation that suits our life-style and personality. Yet as much as the new autonomy is welcomed, it also has its drawbacks. The danger with our freedom of choice is that we may confuse our readiness to mother with our ability to make the "right" choices. In reality, our ability to mother well depends only peripherally on how we resolve these questions. To be ready to mother also requires an emotional and psychological readiness from within.

This book offers little practical help to make the many complex and important decisions mentioned. The real challenge in becoming a mother is to avoid getting so caught up in practical preparations that we forget to pay attention to our inner growth. The best way to prepare for motherhood is thus to attend to the personal transformation.

When does a woman become a mother? Can you really get ready for motherhood in advance? You can look at motherhood strictly as the biological bond between mother and child. In this case, motherhood begins the instant you give birth or sign the adoption papers. Or, you may consider yourself a mother through your actions. You can mother your own or other people's children, or the mental, physical or spiritual needs of other adults, animals, or fauna. Is Mother Theresa a mother? By virtue of her nurturing and caring qualities, she is. Then again, you can be a mother and not exhibit any nurturing qualities. Biologically and legally, you are a mother even if you ignore, abuse, and abandon your child.

Furthermore, we may assume that mothering behaviors are instinctual and appear naturally when a woman gives birth. There is plenty of research evidence for an innate, biological component in mothering. The female hormones, for example, drive the new mother to hold and care for her newborn, albeit fumblingly at first. We may also believe that we already possess the knowledge to mother, because we were mothered ourselves as children. Our past experiences will help us to know what to do as mothers.

These assumptions about the nature of mothering are reassuring to us in pregnancy, when we often feel insecure about our abilities. If it is true that we mother by instinct, then we can relax in pregnancy, knowing that conscious preparation is not necessary. However, as many new mothers attest, motherhood brings such a dramatic change to one's life that any form of preparation in pregnancy will later be appreciated.

Good mothering remains the foundation of every child's well-being. Our society hosts many unmothered children deprived of the foundation for a strong and healthy sense of self. Some of them do not know what it is like to be comforted and soothed when they are in pain. Some do not know what it feels like to be satisfied by just the right amount of food and drink. Some have never been applauded for their achievements. Others have not learned that a firm no can be in their best interest. Few have been allowed to be as teary, messy, mad, or excited as they wanted to be. These children have not had the permission to be themselves.

Unmothered children grow up. Outwardly they may function well as adults. Many find self-esteem by being accomplished and skillful in their chosen careers. Yet they pay the price for their apparently successful adjustment. In order to move forward in life these individuals must bury and hide their inner wounds. They often ridicule and deny their infantile needs and yearnings for the mother they never had. Unconsciously they continue to search for mother and are hurt and disappointed when they do not find her in their adult relationships.

Although not all of us have had a traumatic childhood, our limitations as nurturers are an issue we all face when we become mothers. We are part of a society that has an extremely unrealistic attitude to mothering, in which mothers alternatively are ridiculed and glorified. Women typically escape from this invalidating model of femininity by turning their backs on the nurturing role. We can live happily like this, pursuing our careers and relationships with relative success and letting our nurturing side remain dormant or be channeled into other activities instead. It is not until we want children ourselves that we discover the missing pieces within.

Having collectively abandoned the mothering part of ourselves, we have the potential for emotionally abandoning our children as well. A woman who fails to make a connection to her inner self will have trouble connecting with her child as well. The abandonment is twofold: She deprives both her child and herself of motherly love and care. A true connection between mother and child can only take place when the mother knows who she is. If a woman does not know her true self, she cannot help the child find his.

What are we to do about our conflict-laden relationship toward mothering? We are not helped by turning back and glorifying the past. All was not well when a woman's single purpose in life was to stay home, have children, and become an expert nurturer. Nevertheless, we owe it to our children to be the best mothers we can possibly be. We all know what an important time in one's life childhood is. As mothers-to-be, we cannot escape the issue by saying, "Yes, I know that being a mother is problematic for me, but I will get a good nanny and find the best child care facility in town. My husband will be a good nurturing father for my child. My child does not really need me. He is better off with other caretakers." These arguments are simply excuses that attempt to relieve us of responsibility.

We have to *want to* do the work it takes to become mothers. We must make the commitment, even if we sniff simmering wounds and rotten bones under the surface of our desire to have children. Having a child is a conscious choice these days *and so is becoming a mother.* It is a commitment that carries responsibility to oneself and to one's child.

This is why we must work on our inner transformation in pregnancy. We must learn to protect and care for our deeper needs and aspirations. We must see our potential to abuse, ignore, and abandon ourselves, and thus also our children. When we learn to protect and nurture our soul, we also learn to protect and nurture the soul of our children.

Anna sinks into the rocking chair and lets the motion settle the queasy feeling inside. Here she is again. For three weeks she has known and she still cannot fathom what is happening. Why is her future so hard to imagine? Why can she not see herself as a mother?

Anna rocks steadily back and forth, her eyes closed. She has been so tired lately. She seems to float in and out of a endless dream throughout the day:

Anna steps through the open gate with a pack full of dreams and her sight set on the future. She is ready to follow the path into the thicket. This is a landscape taken by wilderness. Gigantic trees that extend far above her shadow her way. The ground is covered with moss-covered rocks she can stumble upon. A quick glimpse of a white hare—perhaps he will know?—thumping over logs and stones as he disappears into the dark.

The thicket clears and Anna can bask in streams of sunlight until she is ready to see the path continuing into the thicket again. Watch out for spiders, snakes, and swaying shadows wishing to distract you. Do not lose track of your future, do not be late for the child, find the wise woman in the dark, and hurry out of the forest.

Birth! Birth is at the end of the path, the reason she travels so bravely. Then why does she hesitate? Can she not trust? How can she be so close to the miracle of life and yet be oblivious? She cannot stand the upheaval in her womb. She cannot stand the unchanged room she sees from the rocker. Why is the world not changing in response to her findings?

When you are pregnant you are out of your mind. Your rational mind has no choice but to surrender to the surprising moves of your instinctual nature. Body and emotions listen far better to your irrational side than to reason. In this boisterous state of mind you are open to psychological transformation. The fearless, ferocious madwoman within helps you find your new mother-self. You become flexible and formative in your thinking. You find the courage to make the changes, inner as well as outer, that are necessary for you to adapt to motherhood.

Few women are prepared for the haywire state of pregnancy. From what we learn about the physical concerns in the common pregnancy we expect the nine months of gestation to progress, albeit with some discomfort, in a predictable series of events. In the first trimester we anticipate fatigue and nausea; in the second mild edema, occasional dizziness, and constipation; and in the third backaches, frequent urination, and so on.

The emotional and psychological changes can be charted similarly. They progress from the first month of fear and elation; to the subsequent absentmindedness, irritability, and restlessness of the middle months; to the final impatience and excitement of the last month before birth. There is little to suggest that as we step into the pregnant woman's oversized costume we also take on a new, bulky personality.

Facing the wild and crazy psyche can be as scary as facing the fiercest labor pains.

Few women have the courage to meet their feminine madness alone. In this book we will therefore together attempt to discover what this craziness has to do with becoming a mother. It will help you to overcome your inclination to run away in fear. It will suggest ways in which you can explore the uncultivated territory of your inner world. The intention is to teach you to put your inner wilderness to your conscious use. By doing so, you will also learn how to mother your child from that vital inner center.

Anna is going to have a child and it will be a girl. She will have dark brown eyes and long wavy hair so full of luster it will reflect silver specks of moonlight at night. During the day she will run barefoot through sunshine in her petticoat dress on green summer lawns. She will pick yellow dandelions with her little fist and hand the messy bouquet to her mother. She will have a quick temper and a heart as vast as the ocean. Her name will be Miriam.

Anna swallows hard. She cannot get rid of the ill taste in her mouth. In December she will become a mother? Impossible. There must be something she can do. Now. The knot of doubt in her throat is growing. Her hands, seeking reassurance, find her belly.

Pregnancy is the spirit's triumph over reason. Pregnancy can after all not be reduced to an obstetric condition. Life is too grand to remain in the womb. It radiates through Anna's body and besieges her doubts. She is as close to the grandeur of life as she can be. She is pregnant.

In the first months of pregnancy your new mother-self is as shapeless and undeveloped as the fertilized egg in your womb. At this time you may even find it difficult to believe you are pregnant. There are few clear signs to help you recognize what is happening.

As pregnancy proceeds, the physical signs become more pertinent. Your mother-self also leaves the embryonic stage. You initiate a relationship with the primitive, quiet, and unsophisticated human life in your womb. You look for signs of life like the first subtle fluttering in your abdomen, and as you become aware of your child's presence he begins to come alive to you. Your behavior matches the inner changes you experience. It is obvious to everyone that you are pregnant, not only by how you look, but what you do and what you talk about.

In the last months of pregnancy the baby takes more and more room in body and mind alike. You engage in small talk with your unborn child; you wonder about his looks and his likes, his temper and talents; and most of all you want to know when you will finally meet. At this point, having a child on your mind is natural. Motherhood is near.

The experiences in pregnancy are particularly important for women who find it difficult to envision themselves as mothers. For whatever reason a woman doubts her abilities; whether it be because of the emotional wounds of her upbringing or because she rejects the traditional mother role or simply because she does not consider herself particularily nurturing as a woman, she must work through her anxieties during this time. If she can stay with the psychological process as it unfolds in pregnancy, she will gradually develop an inner source to turn to for advice and reassurance in her mothering role.

To be full of yourself, as self-conscious and self-centered as you wish, is a privilege of pregnancy. Once you give birth there will be little time and energy left for such indulgences. We usually think of egocentrism as the antithesis of good mothering. A mother who is self-absorbed thinks only of her own needs and ignores her children's. It may thus seem that encouraging self-consciousness in pregnancy denies the need for us to be generous and altruistic as mothers. Would we not prepare ourselves better for this task if we began setting ourselves aside and concentrated on the child in the womb instead?

Ignoring ourselves does not make us better mothers. Our self-preoccupation serves an important function: By nourishing and protecting our own psychological transformation we learn to nurture the developing self of the child as well. When we attend to our own needs and wishes we attain confidence and inner direction we need to care genuinely for our children.

Although you have been instructed to prepare for motherhood, you will now be advised to do nothing of the sort. All you have to do is to be pregnant. Find a place low in the abdomen, close to your child, and let yourself receive. Be as open as you can to whatever comes along, and your experiences will enter and work you inside out. Pregnancy will stir and shake you; it will loosen and tighten, soften and strengthen you where it is needed. Pregnancy will make you a mother.

To say that you should do nothing but be open and receptive to your experiences in pregnancy does not mean that you can get lazy and let the nine months pass over your head. Staying put and protected in your abdomen takes conscious work. If you forget, the outer world will soon take over and become your only teacher about motherhood. You are part of the culture you live in, and you cannot and should not avoid listening to what is expected from you as a mother. But if you follow only what society tells you is true, you will look well adjusted from the outside, doing what has been taught to you and winning the approval of others, but you will become a mother only superficially. You will not have done the inner work necessary to become a mother at heart.

We cannot pick out the areas of the transformation we are comfortable with or interested in and skip the ones that bore us and make us anxious. If you prefer to contemplate the profound meaning of motherhood and make this the focus of pregnancy you will be ill prepared for the reality of diaper changes and breast engorgement when pregnancy is over. Your new insights mean nothing when you have to give your newborn his first bath or pin on a diaper for the first time. Preparing yourself for motherhood involves being equally ready to absorb the minute details of infant care and the recondite and heartfelt.

How will you find her, the mother within, whom no one else can introduce you to? Will you find her in the doctor's office or with a midwife? Will she be introduced to you in a parenting course? Perhaps she is personified in someone you know? Does she bear any resemblance to your own mother or some other woman you admire? Since she is of your own flesh and blood, will a genetic consultation help?

The mother you are looking for will not appear to you suddenly and in her full glory. She will not come to you; you must take the trouble to search for her. You will have to gather proof of her existence one piece at a time: Look for her shadow as it falls on the ground; follow her fading footprints in the wet sand; find the places where her smell lingers, a seat still warm from her body heat, a creation she has nurtured to bloom. See what she has brought to life and what she has left untouched. Look for her children, young and old. You will find her presence everywhere.

Forget about how you normally comprehend matters. Your chances of finding the mother within are better if you leave your mind alone and let your senses guide you. What parts of your body know her best? Can you feel a tingle, a shiver, or a warm rush when she is present? Let her breath mingle with yours. Eat of her rich and savory food. Take her in at a pace you are able to digest. Slowly but surely you will include her when you think about yourself as a mother.

It is important to find your own private sanctuary where you can nourish your emerging mother-self. This will be the place you turn to when you wish to focus your energy on your transformation. Here you can reflect on the many changes you are facing; you can clarify your ideas and visualize the future.

There are many ways to explore and contemplate your thoughts and feelings about motherhood. For some, *journaling* is their preferred way to articulate thoughts and feelings. Writing allows you to balance your intuitive side, which uses images and symbols to express and understand, with your rational side, which uses logic to analyze and organize your experiences. The word *diary* means "a book of days." Writing in your diary is an easy way to make sure you keep the inner process going through all the days of pregnancy. The diary produces material you can return to again and again, perhaps finding new meanings each time. Over time your journal becomes a written account of your transformation to mother.

For others, *dreams* are important. Dreams are a rich source of material for exploring our reactions to motherhood. They can be understood as allegories that contain messages from our unconscious. The different characters in a dream play out our conflicting feelings and ideas. Our fears and desires thus get a chance to emerge uncensored. Dreams also transcend the limits of time and space that our rational mind imposes on our thoughts. They give us a chance to try out our mother-self before we give birth.

Poetry is another way of exploring your experiences in pregnancy. The condensed and spare format of a poem provides a powerful way to clarify ideas and express the feelings that are the essence of the transformation to mother.

If your *artistic talents* are more pronounced than your verbal skills, you may choose to work with, for example, clay, watercolors, or textile. Artwork can reveal meanings and express a depth of feeling that words fail to convey. As symbolic representations, they speak directly from the soul. Art also speaks *to* our soul. Even if we are not artistically inclined we can deepen our understanding of motherhood by looking at the art of others.

Some enjoy exploring internal matters in the company of others and prefer to seek out other expecting parents in a *discussion group*. Sharing your different experiences of pregnancy with others is a stimulating and thought-provoking way of working on your transformation. It is reassuring to see how we all struggle with similar issues in pregnancy. Giving and receiving empathy and care helps you gain the support and confidence you need in becoming a mother.

As we have seen, there are many ways to let your inner self tell you about motherhood. Whichever media you choose for your explorations, there are a few conditions to remember:

Let your mind play with as few constrictions as possible. A set agenda will only block access to your inner self. Allow your thoughts to flow freely and spontaneously. Let them be chaotic. Let them appear and disappear as they please. Use as little structure as possible. Let your thoughts dance their own spontaneous dance in your mind. The object is to let your inner self surprise, stir, and confuse you.

Trust your process. Only when you can accept whatever comes along will you be gifted with new insights. The meaning will appear to you in due course. You will know what you have done when you are done. Harvesting is done when the crop is ready.

Be honest with yourself. If you allow yourself to find out what you really feel, want, and believe, you will discover who you really are. Do not expect your new mother-self to be static. In pregnancy we are evolving and changing so rapidly that it is difficult to find continuity and consistency in the self-image.

Ambivalence is natural in any transformative process. We want and fear the changes at the same time. The more daring you become in reaching the deep recesses of your inner self, the more aware you will be of the paradoxical nature of your thoughts and feelings. When you can allow them to surface without judgment you learn to appreciate how multifaceted the mothering role will be.

Chapter 1

PROJECT BABY

As Thomas grasps Anna's hand, a soft overture of electronic beeps breaks their silence. A flickering white light fills the dark screen in front of them. The picture stabilizes as the camera lens sweeps across a foreign scene. It is a view lacking in details: vast, barren areas in different shades of gray, dimly separated from each other by winding borders. Can this be other than a desolate world?

"Here on the left side is one of the kidneys," says the technician at their side. "A little larger than normal, but this is common in pregnancy. I am just going to change frequency, and then you will see."

Anna and Thomas stare intently at the screen. There! This is what they have been waiting for. They have seen enough pictures in the books to know what to look for. Hiding in the corner is a tiny little being, not larger than a thumb, curled up like the ampersand symbol, "&." Unbelievable! Little "&," floating freely like a balloon in the dark space of the womb, securely fastened to a sturdy-looking cord. How bravely alone she is in this world that does not distinguish between night and day. Looking so peacefully unaware, can she possibly sense she is being observed?

"My little baby, you are so beautiful!"

"This is incredible!"

" Eyes as large as blueberries, but I think they must be brown."

"A good-sized brain and a big heart."

"You have your father's stooping legs."

"And your mother's vacant look."

"Look, she moved!"

"Probably shy. Too much attention at once."

"So athletic."

"Is that little thing there a penis?"

The lab technician, clearing her throat, interrupts them. She is done with her measurements, she says. Would they like a snapshot to take home?

Anna attaches the blurred photo to the refrigerator door so they can look at it many times a day. It is proof that her pregnancy is not just a fantasy she shares with Thomas, but the beginning of a human life—their child.

"I am sure now. It is actually going to happen. I am carrying a child," she declares.

Seeing the fetus on the ultrasound scan has finally convinced her. Besides, when she runs her hands over her stomach she can feel it is starting to bulge in a novel shape. Things are starting to happen, and they are happening fast. Anna feels restless.

"I must get ready," she thinks. "I am already behind schedule."

When you start recognizing the first human characteristics of your growing fetus, perhaps feeling it move, hearing its heartbeat, or seeing it on a sonogram, it is an exciting moment. All of a sudden the few lingering doubts that you are carrying a life fade. Even at this early stage the fetus is unmistakably human. It is kicking and turning, generating its own audible heartbeat, and already signaling its uniqueness in the finest details, like the web of vessels covering the eyelids or the skinfolds crisscrossing the palms. It is no longer so hard to imagine holding a baby in your arms.

At this time the need to prepare seems more urgent than it did in the very beginning of pregnancy. But what can you really do to get ready for motherhood at this early point?

One Saturday afternoon when the rain taps the windows Anna sits down in front of her bookcase and clears out all her paperback classics from the top shelf. Lawrence, Woolf, and Hemingway have to go—even her favorite Atwood collection. Fiction has to give way to non-fiction; the topics are pregnancy, parenting, and children. These brand new books with their matter-of-fact language evoke the same curiosity and excitement as the most captivating novel. The written word will initiate her into the world of parenthood.

One by one Anna leans the titles against the bookends. First, the books on pregnancy. She has two of them, and she has read every page many times. Then come the books on infant care, yet to be opened. She finds her book on nursing and places it in between the others. How fascinating to see an entire book devoted to explaining how babies eat, she thinks. She takes the four dry but important-looking books on children's growth and development, and adds to them a handeddown copy of Dr. Spock and glistening new copies of books by Penelope Leach and Dr. Berry Brazelton, two modern gurus on parenting. Then comes a thick volume on childhood diseases, which she knows she will never dare to open. Finally she places a pile of old copies of Mothering *magazine on the shelf and props up a manila folder with handouts from the doctor's office.*

Anna steps back and looks at what she has accomplished. Neatly arranged on the shelf are all her hopes for the future. A long string of letters, words, lines, and pages forms the answer to the mystery of motherhood. Will they keep their promise and offer her their wisdom?

Like Anna, as you try to get a grip on motherhood, what first comes to your mind is to gather as much information as possible. Excitedly, you set out on a hunt for baby literature, audiotapes and videotapes, and anything else you can get your hands on. There is no shortage of material. From the very beginning of pregnancy, mothers-to-be are showered with books, pamphlets, magazines, videos, and invitations to lectures, all offering advice on the best ways to parent. They cover everything from the down-to-earth matters of nutrition, hygiene, childhood diseases, and what baby items to buy to the complexity of what constitutes the most favorable emotional and educational environment.

Reading about babies is fun. When the due date seems far away, it is nice to resort to magazines and books filled with charming baby pictures to nourish your curiosity and excitement about the future. At the same time the sincere wish to become the best parent possible is taken care of. Up-to-date knowledge is important when you want to make wise decisions for your child. Additionally, for many, studying the subject is their only way to find out about babies. Not everyone has had the opportunity for close contact with children. And for those who have seen other parents struggle with their young ones, the need to meet the challenge wellprepared may seem even more important.

As the good mother you wish to become, you bravely dive into the subject matter.

Becoming a mother is the most extensive project Anna has ever aimed for. She is preparing herself to take care of a fragile human life, a task that is not to be taken lightly. It requires her to be responsible, mature, and of sound judgment. Anna has convinced herself that she now is ready for this demanding project. She may not know anything about motherhood yet, but she sure knows how to find out. Knowledge is the key, and as she has done ever since school and in her jobs she will just have to learn what she does not know. Finding out about motherhood is no different. She knows exactly how to approach this new mission—her Project Baby.

She has already taken the first step. She has gathered as many facts about babies as she can. Her collection of books has replaced her ignorance with a rather substantial awareness of little ones and what they need. The next step will be to sort out the myriad pieces of advice she has found. This will not be easy. There is so much out there, and the experts often contradict each other. Some sources claim, for instance, that it is best to nurse whenever the infant cries, whereas others say that establishing a feeding pattern is important for the baby's comfort. What should she believe? And what is she to do with all the words of wisdom she receives from experienced mothers? How do they compare to the elegant theories of the experts? And what about the baby magazines? Are they reliable or not?

The questions are countless. Yet, if she just uses her wit she will be able to sort out the pros and cons of the many alternatives. Then all she will have to do is to determine which option will be the very best for her child. This important step will require all of her analytical abilities, a sound judgment, as well as some good old common sense. Then, "Voila!" She will have found the perfect way to mother Miriam, and by this time Project Baby will produce a real baby!

Most of us will use a systematic, methodical strategy to handle our questions about motherhood. Such an approach comes naturally for women of the nineties, many of us who have let careers precede childbearing. We are quick to apply the same skills needed in the workplace to pregnancy: decisiveness, organization, and preparation. Using the same routine as we would with any job assignment, we set out to tackle Project Baby with all the enthusiasm summoned for this very important experience in life. We gather ample information, learn the proper techniques, plan the future in detail, and make all the important decisions we think are needed to bring our vision of parenthood alive. Accordingly, many women today approach motherhood in a rational, judicious manner. We concentrate on the practical skills required for the task.

This professionalized approach is not novel to us. It is how our high-tech society works. We demand specialization and proficiency in most areas of activity. Motherhood is no different. Just look at what we meet in pregnancy. Science has forever changed our ideas of how babies are made from a tale of stork deliveries to a complex technological procedure. We are now familiar with a vocabulary of terms like "invitro fertilization," "alpha-fetoprotein tests," and "amniocentesis." For each of these procedures there is at least one high-tech instrument and one specialist. With such complex possibilities to begin and to monitor pregnancy we set equally high expectations for dealing with the result of our efforts. If pregnancy can be manipulated into the microcosm of sperm and egg cells, surely what the real baby will do can be similarily controlled? For successful parenting we will just follow the same formula of listening to the experts and taking advantage of their latest advancements.

So prolific and fascinating is the field of infancy that we can easily spend the whole pregnancy engrossed in the subject. Our efforts make us a generation of wellinformed parents, but is learning all the practical how-tos really all that motherhood is about? We do not have to spend many minutes with a child to realize that book knowledge is not enough to deal with a lively spirit. Children will not be satisfied with less than our total involvement, including attention, patience, wit, and the last drop of energy. There is nothing like experience to provide what it takes, but this is certainly a poor comfort to the first-time mother. How, then, can we compensate for our inexperience without falling prey to hypothetical nonsense?

The nine months of pregnancy offer plenty of opportunity to prepare for the psychological as well as the practical side of motherhood. In order to accomplish this you need to set aside Project Baby and turn your attention to the main character of motherhood-yourself. Whereas the former is an extroverted activity that keeps your focus on the material and away from yourself, paying attention to how you are changing as a person is introverted work. As such, it does not follow the logical, step-by-step procedure learning about babies does. Instead it challenges you to make use of your emotions and intuition as well as your mind creatively. The purpose is not to learn how to mother, but to help you start thinking about yourself as a mother.

In this chapter we will examine both the practical and the psychological approach to learning about motherhood. First we will talk more about our intellectual preparations illustrated by Project Baby. We will see just what we expect to know as mothers and where we get these notions from. We will ask how our trust in the advice of experts affects us as new mothers. Later on, we will learn more about the inner emotional growth in pregnancy and see what we can do to encourage it.

OUR SCIENTIFIC VIEW OF PARENTING

We live in a society based on an extensive interchange of facts and information, a modern circumstance of life that extends even to new parents. Gone are the days when it was assumed that all that was needed to raise a child were your motherly instinct and common sense. Instead we have inherited an awareness of children's needs brought to our attention by the specialists in the field of human development. We believe in the goodness and helpfulness of absorbing their research findings and instructions.

Scientific knowledge shapes our expectations of what we need to do to become decent parents. In addition to possessing a pound of loving and caring, as parents we should know about children's motor, cognitive, emotional, and social development. Most handbooks on parenting have extensive tables of exactly what your child is supposed to be doing each month and what you can do to encourage his or her development. We eagerly devour this material. Parenting looks so reassuringly simple on paper. If we just follow the advice given, we will have the intelligent, happy, and welladjusted children we hoped for.

What, then, are some of the beliefs about children we adhere to, and who are the authorities telling us what is important to know? Let us take a look at some common ideas about what good parents do and try to find their origins and current supporters.

"Good parents turn to professionals for answers to their questions"
The trust we put in "the scientific child-rearing method," that is, our willingness to turn to experts for advice on what to do with our children, can be traced back to the beginning of the century when the scholarly interest in children's behavior arose. Scientists like John B. Watson and B. F. Skinner of the behaviorist tradition claimed it was possible to shape the character of humans if you only followed their elaborate methods of controlling the nursery environment and the parents' interactions with their children. All parents had to do to determine what their children would become, Watson and Skinner implied, was simply manipulate what their young ones were exposed to.

Since then more pragmatic behaviorists have produced many practical handbooks on how to shape children's behavior. Concepts of modern parenting jargon (like "time out" and "positive and negative reinforcement") are based on the principles of behaviorism. For example, the book *Parent Effectiveness Training* by Dr. Thomas Gordon[1] has had great impact on child rearing practices and is often recommended by psychologists. In simple and straightforward terms, he instructs parents how to act with their children. Gordon's easily comprehended "how-to" approach is intended to help empower parents when children are out of control.

The behaviorist tradition promoted the idea that parents might not automatically know how to parent and might need to acquire parenting skills. Thus good parenting is viewed as a premeditated, deliberate, and informed activity. But this approach is not without problems. If carried to the extreme, the determinism inherent in the theory implies that because parents shape their children's personalities, they are also responsible for any undesirable behaviors the children exhibit. It is the parents' fault when the little ones have problems. Although parents unquestionably have great impact on their children's development, such theoretical dogma exaggerates the anxieties and self-doubts that normally plague the new parent.

"Good parents provide their children with intellectual stimulation"
There has been a great deal of research into infant cognitive development, much of which has filtered down to parents. Most of us have heard about Jean Piaget's theory of cognitive development, which proposes that a child's intellectual development follows a fixed sequence. From Piaget's theory, and the related field of research on human intelligence, we gather many suggestions about how we can provide our children with the appropriate intellectual stimulation at the appropriate time. Some of these research findings have found their way into the nursery, as can be seen in the black and white mobiles parents hang over a baby's crib to catch the attention of the color-insensitive newborn.

"Good parents bond with their children"
From the psychodynamic tradition, with Freud as the forefather and later represented by Erik Erikson, Anna Freud, and Margaret Mahler among others, comes the emphasis on children's emotional development. They have taught us that childhood experiences determine our mental health as adults and particularly that the early relationship between mother and child is important.

We have adopted a number of expressions from their theories, which we fondly use when we talk about parenting. "Bonding" is one such popularized concept. We ascribe the greatest importance to it and give it an almost magical quality. Mothers talk about setting aside time for bonding, as if it is possible to control exactly when and how the close relationship between mother and child will develop. This is a good example of how we tend to complicate the most natural aspects of motherhood with semiscientific jargon. In the case of bonding, we might as well say that it is important to spend time with our children for them to feel secure.

The emphasis in psychodynamic theory on the child's first year gives rise to much concern in new mothers. The fear that we will fail in this fundamental task creeps into everyday dilemmas like feeding and sleeping habits: What happens if I do not offer the breast when my child cries? Should the baby sleep in our bed or not? Can I let him cry himself to sleep or not? Finding the right balance between the infant's preferences and ours is a difficult task. We should certainly be sensitive to the needs of our children, but at some point we must set limits on what we are willing to do or we will have nothing left to give.

These are only a few of the many current credos on parenting. Knowledge of the many different expert opinions is a mixed blessing. It is nice for novices to have solid advice to follow, yet it can also seem that parenthood is only suitable for reputable specialists. Who would have ever thought our child's first days of life would be such a complex matter? Measured against how much there is to know, our limited knowledge appears hopelessly inadequate. We often wish we could return to the golden age of our grandmothers: The less there was to learn, the less there was to confuse us.

By implication all theories convey the same message: As a parent you are responsible for your child's development—your very words, gestures, emotions, and attitudes shape who he or she will become. Is it then so strange if we think we must learn to parent to perfection and feel hopelessly inadequate when we fail? Looking to the ideals of fanciful theories to see what is expected of us is certainly a hard way to learn about motherhood.

Most of the information available to parents is oriented toward the baby and its needs and does not tell them what it is like to be a mother or a father. Specialists who present their ideas from the child's perspective have a hard time conveying any support for the other party—that is, for the parent. Being left alone with your own needs and concerns puts enormous pressure on you in a situation that is strenuous in itself. As a new parent you need support rather than intimidation, whether it comes from understanding friends, family, or professionals, or from self-help books that acknowledge the difficulties.

As we have seen, it is easy to feel overwhelmed and insecure when you are presented with an abundance of information. How, then, are these uncomfortable feelings handled? Although it may seem better to stay away from intimidating educational material, paradoxically many of us tackle our self-doubts by embarking on a hectic quest for increasingly more child care information. We convince ourselves that if only we finish the fifth book on breast-feeding, the annoying uncertainty about our nursing abilities will disappear.

After this array of unfortunate consequences, we must remember that our intellectual pursuits are not only a defensive reaction to the hardship we foresee but also a very helpful way to prepare. Intellectual preparations will bridge the transition between the present life-style and motherhood. As you read about parenting and children, you gain practice in thinking like a parent, albeit on a hypothetical level. In the wonderful world of your imagination, you can picture the world's most beautiful child and ask yourself how you would care for it. You can try different alternatives and make sure to find the perfect solutions to the most intricate problems, all while the child in your body is safely unaware of your experiments.

Although a constructed way of understanding what it means to be a mother, taking a rational approach is the best we can do until parenthood becomes a reality. The danger is that we become so caught up in this mode of thinking that it becomes our only way of dealing with the adjustment. There are limits to how far this form of intellectual preparation can take us. As we shall see, in many ways, Project Baby *does not* completely prepare us for the future.

HOW PROJECT BABY MISLEADS US

". . . and by this time Project Baby will produce a real baby!" Produce? Anna suddenly realizes Miriam might have one or two objections if she could utter any words. To be regarded as a product is not very flattering. Indeed, she could be the

product of a very ambitious and well-planned project, but this is little comfort. After all, a product is an object, and as such it has neither soul nor will. It would not be much fun to see your parents anxiously watching your every move to find evidence for success with their little product. If you did something good, they would credit themselves for having chosen the right method. If, however, you messed up, they would panic over their catastrophic miscalculation or blame themselves for not yet having perfected their chosen method.

No, Anna has to be careful not to carry her baby project too far. Still, she really wants to be a carefully prepared and informed mother. If she could trust she knows enough to avoid the worst mistakes in raising her child, she could relax. Maybe she would even enjoy being a mother!

When you depend on your rational mind alone to learn how to be a mother, you have the illusion that everything a mother faces can be easily controlled. If Project Baby runs smoothly according to plan, then surely you think it is a good indication of how you will act as a parent. Yet being in control is rarely your first experience when you are getting acquainted with your new baby. The differences in size and life experience between the two of you do not seem to have anything to do with who is in charge. In spite of your apparent superiority, you will nevertheless not be able to decide when you want your child to eat, sleep, cry, or smile. When your most sincere attempts fail, it is hard not to feel both incompetent and frustrated.

Similarly, in pregnancy you are free to use your nine months of preparation any way you want. There may be certain things you wish to accomplish, but when and how you make your preparations for birth are up to you. Having an infant will put an end to this freedom. You will now have to get used to following the rhythm of your baby instead of your own, a rhythm that is both exhausting and unpredictable.

Taking full responsibility for your baby project in pregnancy comes naturally. After all, it is your parental duty to make sure your baby gets the best kind of treatment you can provide. Caring for a real baby is a different matter. It is all too easy to feel responsible for events you cannot change. You may feel guilty when your baby has a hard day, when she is below average on the growth chart, when she catches a cold, and so on, for a million factors. Learning what you are responsible for and what is beyond your control is, as in life at large, difficult.

The chaos of the first weeks, a very emotional time, may come as a surprise. You have probably read all about what to expect in your baby books, and because you have seen it in print you believe you are prepared for the tumult. Yet reading about being exhausted and feeling down is somehow not the same as experiencing it. It is still so difficult to handle. All of a sudden your old ways of handling stressful situations no longer work, and you must struggle to find new ways of coping.

Project Baby can also mislead you into believing that you do not have to change much to become a parent. You may try to plan your future with the baby in detail. You imagine how he or she will fit in like the missing piece to complete the giant jigsaw puzzle of your life. You see no need to change when and how you relate to your partner and friends, when you work, play, and do whatever else fills your days. It is hard to understand that, especially in the beginning, it is you who will have to adjust your life to your child and not the other way around.

In reality motherhood does not follow the same predictable course as its mental equivalent does. And thank goodness for that. For the person who has trained herself to follow the logical structure of her rational mind, motherhood opens up a whole new dimension of being. If you are used to thinking about your time in terms of accomplishments and goals, spending the days with your nonscheming baby will set you off in a different direction. You are free to discover what happens when you sit back and let the time spent with your baby unfold itself. Where sober distance and objectivity used to be essential qualities, now you can lose yourself in intense involvement and emotionality. Who cares about getting anything done when you have the world's most wonderful baby in your arms?

YOUR EMOTIONS DURING PREGNANCY AND HOW THEY PREPARE YOU FOR MOTHERHOOD

It is a tepid summer evening. The air carries a heavy scent of sweet jasmine and fresh-cut grass, mixed with the rancid smell of popcorn and pizza. Music, laughter, and cries rise toward the darkening sky. People stroll happily down the crowded paths. The lines are long in front of the concession stands and lottery booths. It is the perfect night to visit the old amusement park. Anna loves this place. It throws her back to a time when a new balloon and a ride on the merry-go-round would send her into ecstasy. Anna takes a deep breath. There are a lot of people out tonight. Many elbows touch her. Kids whine for candy. A gang of teenagers sway in front of her. One of them, a red-faced, sulleneyed youngster, burps sour beer in her face. Anna feels faint. She grabs Thomas's arm. He smiles and gives her a quick kiss. In front of them a large woman in a Mexican sun hat cuts out and targets Anna's stomach with her swaying arm.

"Watch out. Damn it. You bitch!" Anna hears herself shouting. The woman does not notice. She has already entered the gambling arcade. Thomas looks at Anna, his brown eyes glistening.

"What's the matter?"

"Nothing."

Tears pour down Anna's flashing hot cheeks. She starts to run, zigzagging her way through the crowd, bumping into a toddler in his stroller, tripping over an empty flowerpot. She hears Thomas shouting from behind, but she does not stop. Colors, faces, lights swirl around her. She must find a place to sit. There is an empty bench next to the concert hall entrance and she throws herself down on it. She clutches her hands around her knees to stop herself from trembling. Her pulse is racing. Thomas catches up with her.

"What's the matter?" he asks again.

"I want to go home," Anna sobs. "I hate this place."

Strong, turbulent feelings reign in pregnancy. They indicate the magnitude of the adjustment the pregnant woman is going through. As well as being a natural reaction to the physical and psychological demands of carrying a child, these emotional ups and downs appear in response to the inner psychological transformation that is taking place. Accepting the new mother-self is as much an emotional as a mental process. The mother-to-be needs the nine months of pregnancy to express and sort out the feelings elicited.

When we get caught up in the many facts and practical details of Project Baby it is easy to forget the emotional labor needed in pregnancy. After all, feelings lack the reassuring certainty academic baby knowledge has. They are much more nebulous, arbitrary, and difficult to comprehend. Often we are left alone to handle them. It is fairly easy to find help for the practical problems we face as inexperienced mothers, but rarely do we get help to prepare for the shower of feelings the arrival of the baby will bring. The health practitioners are more concerned with the physical health of mother and child, and they spend little time discussing the subjective experience of mothering. Our own mothers have conveniently forgotten what it was like in the beginning, and other mother-friends often keep quiet, perhaps in an effort to protect either us or themselves.

Mothering is one of the most impassioned experiences a woman can have in her lifetime. As an activity, it requires her full emotional involvement. In most other feats she can choose to set aside her feelings for the moment if intellect, endurance, or concentration is more crucial to accomplish her goals; but she cannot mother in this fashion. A child needs his mother to be emotionally available during his awake hours. The mother must set aside her other worries so she can give freely to her child. At the same time, the feelings he awakens in her are of a seldom encountered intensity. They run deep, raw, and fervent. Aside from heavenly love and happiness, there are feelings that are hard to reconcile, such as resentment, envy, vengefulness, or sorrow.

Motherhood can be so bewildering that the difficulties overshadow the joys. Yet, for the woman who impatiently awaits the arrival of her child, the idea of having mixed feelings when the baby finally arrives seems odd or outright unsound. She is sure the wondrous gift of a newborn child will make her nothing but exuberant and grateful. Understandably, she is reluctant to look at the opposite side of maternal bliss.

Recently, in an attempt to break the silence surrounding the subject, several authors have addressed the fact that motherhood is a perplexing experience, far from the ceaseless gratification so many women expect. Books such as *Motherhood: What It Does to Your Mind,*[2] *The Myth of the Bad Mother,*[3] and *The New Mother Syndrome*[4] speak of the conflictual situations and emotional duress mothers experience. These books are not always pleasant reading, because we all would like to believe in the unmixed happiness the child will bring. Yet, only when the other emotions of motherhood are openly discussed can we get past the shame and guilt over these feelings that isolate and incapacitate, and begin looking for ways to alleviate the pressure on new mothers.

MOTHERHOOD BRINGS A NEW LIFE AND NEW FEELINGS

What is it about becoming a mother that makes it such a tumultuous experience? As a major life event it will affect practically all aspects of your life. First, there are the sobering conditions under which you are left to cope with your new family member. Physically, you will be exhausted after nine months of hard body work, crowned by labor and delivery. The hormonal fluctuations associated with postpartum recovery and lactation render you emotionally unstable, often as close to tears as to exhilaration. Added to these physical factors are the stresses of adjusting to the new role. As a new parent you are a beginner struggling to learn how to care for the baby. Understanding the subtle signals of an infant is not effortless, nor is nursing, changing diapers, or bathing him. You and your spouse will have to decide on how to share these responsibilities. You will also have to work out a new relationship between you with somewhat new rules for how to interact. Furthermore, you must redirect your energy from the outside world to home, which may mean giving up activities you enjoy, losing the daily support of work companions, and facing the all-too-common isolation at home. All of these changes give rise to a multitude of feelings that need attention.

Emotions also abound when expectations are not met. You find out that feeding and changing diapers on a twenty-four-hour basis is tedious and repetitive work. The darling infant whose big achievement of the day is to focus on the stripes of his mother's shirt is not intellectually stimulating. You get bored and wish you could escape to more exciting company. You envy your childless friends who are free to take off as they please. You feel disappointed, frustrated, remorseful. It is equally disturbing to realize that you also fail to be as good a mother as your child deserves. The baby boy cries miserably and you cannot figure out why; a forgotten diaper change gives the poor guy a rash; you take him to a party where he is exposed to germs that cause his first cold, and so on. We all believe that mothers should not make mistakes that hurt their children; mothers should not feel lonely, irritated, bored, or vindictive; yet we do, and it is very upsetting.

HOW YOU CAN WORK WITH YOUR FEELINGS IN PREGNANCY

What is the matter with Anna? She is as volatile as a spring afternoon: At first she is sunny and bright, but dark clouds hover at the horizon, and before you know it a fierce hailstorm hammers her freckled skin. A lightning bolt crosses the sky and furious thunder soon shakes the neighborhood. Then silence. Before long the sun is there again, soothing the frightened blossoms.

"It is like you have swallowed a burning log," Thomas says. "You look so innocent, but then you open your mouth and roaring flames come out."

Anna does not know herself anymore. She cannot predict her own moves. They will be dramatic, certainly, and sentimental, but that is all she knows. Her unpredictability is exciting and disturbing at the same time.

"I guess you cannot help it," Thomas says. "It's what happens when women get pregnant."

"Don't patronize me!" Anna bursts out. "You are reducing me to a hormonal condition. I am who I am. I just happen to have a lot of feelings."

Is there something we can do to prepare ourselves so that the kick into the reality of motherhood will not be so harsh? Yes there is, as long as we understand that we cannot escape our emotions. We are living, feeling beings and will therefore experience love and happiness as well as anger, confusion, and gloom as we learn to cope with our new existence. Pregnancy prepares us for what is coming. The many emotions of this eventful time serve as a guide into motherhood. As we learn about ourselves from our reactions to pregnancy, we simultaneously prepare for what awaits us as new mothers. We learn what makes us comfortable and confident and what brings us down. We find that feelings can grab us and take us into deep waters, but also that there are ways to get out of them. The experience of pregnancy thus allows us to experience the whole palette of emotions but not be overwhelmed by them.

But how do our feelings during pregnancy relate to motherhood, of which we yet know so little? To understand, we must remember that the transition into motherhood is a process of personal growth that spans both pregnancy and the first few months with the baby. It takes time to become familiar with and find ways to express what you are going through and then to understand and work through these feelings. The earlier you pay attention to your emotional reactions to this process, the easier it will be to cope after the baby is born.

How can you use the feelings you have at present to prepare you for the early months with the baby? A good starting point is to get acquainted with your typical reactions to change. Certainly, there is no lack of opportunities. There is your first response when you find out that you are pregnant. There is the time you realize you are treated differently by others now that you are expecting. You may face physical complications or at least the possibility of them. You must get used to being bigger, more tired, and less productive. The concluding event is also the most dramatic—giving birth. All these situations affect you one way or another. You may kick and scream, soak your pillow with tears, or try to ignore the existence of any disturbing feelings. Whatever your reactions may be, they are worth reflecting upon.

Try holding on to your feelings for a while, even when they make you uneasy. Ask yourself how familiar they are, and how comfortable you are with them. Can you tolerate them or do you instantly chase them away? When pregnancy makes you react in new and unfamiliar ways, you may become concerned. It is tempting to try to push the feelings away and that may be wise when they threaten to overwhelm you; but if you succeed, they are likely to return with even greater intensity once the child is born. At this time, you also have the baby to care for, and you will have much less time and energy for yourself.

It is also common to be judgmental about your feelings. "Is this really normal?" you may ask. "Why am I behaving so strangely? Is this really how pregnant women feel? The joy leaves nothing to worry about, but what about the other feelings? I am supposed to be happy, but why do these embarrassing thoughts of not liking motherhood one bit creep up underneath the excitement?" When self-reproach follows these doubts your self-confidence can shrink to a tiny speck. It is important to affirm your feelings and not reject or condemn them. If you can begin the process of accepting and coping with them during pregnancy, it is easier to face the difficult moments of motherhood with humor and forgiveness.

Try to understand what your emotions have to tell you about yourself and your needs. Is it enough to know that you are reacting in a normal way to a new and stressful situation? Do you need someone to talk to, someone who can reassure you that you will get through to the other side? Do you need a plan of action? If you take care of your emotional needs during pregnancy, you will be more able to know what kind of support you will need after you give birth, and you will make sure that support will be available.

There are some concrete questions you must ask yourself. First, how are you going to vent your frustrations and replenish your energies as a mother? Who will be there to relieve you? How will you and your partner share the responsibilities? Mothering can tire and frustrate you just as pregnancy does, and you need to find ways to restore your well-being. Second, how will you find an outlet for your ambitions and creativity? Where will you find intellectual stimulation? When will you have adult company? How can you stay physically fit? Most of us mistakenly believe the baby will satisfy these needs, but it is the satisfaction of getting your own needs met that will sustain you in mothering him or her.

It is sometimes useful to try to get a deeper understanding of why we react in a certain way. This task can be complex and ensnaring because we are not always consciously aware of the origin of our feelings. Unresolved conflicts from the past, which color present experiences, may be at work. These conflicts may affect the ease of adjusting to motherhood. According to a study by Dr. Ann Frodi at the University of Rochester,[5] pregnant women who had painful and unresolved experiences during their childhood reacted more negatively to infant cries than others. As mothers, they more frequently perceived their children as difficult to care for although there was no observable evidence that the children were more difficult. Unfortunately, for these women the feelings lingering from the past make mothering more difficult. It is even more important for these women to get support, both in caring for the child and in unraveling the past.

THE DIFFICULT FEELINGS OF PREGNANCY AND HOW THEY RELATE TO MOTHERHOOD

Anna cannot forget the evening at the amusement park. It frightens her to think about it. Somewhere in the cheerful crowd, among the spinning wheels, lottery booths, and merry-go-rounds, she lost herself. She revisits the park in her dream. Soon the cascade of feelings tears through her like flashing fireworks. She sees herself climbing aboard the old wooden roller coaster. She sits alone in the last car. The train takes off. It climbs a long hill and shoots into the darkness on the other side. It careens up, down, and through the turns at higher and higher speed. Anna's eyes start to water and she feels sick. She shouts to the driver to slow down, but he does not listen. He, or perhaps it is a she, is only about three inches tall and cannot reach the brakes anyway. She pulls the string that runs between them. The driver inflates to a balloon and rises merrily to the sky. She is left alone to circle the loop of her inner turmoil.

Having no control over a situation is one of the most anxiety-provoking experiences we can encounter. We need to feel we have power over both our inner and outer worlds in order to be at ease. As discussed earlier, the stresses of having a new baby will likely trigger such feelings at first. Now think about what it is like to be pregnant. Do you perhaps already feel out of control at times? Dramatic mood swings may send you on your own roller-coaster ride. Your body reacts in new ways. You are no longer sure of who you are. Unfamiliar situations, such as going through medical procedures that have not been explained, trigger these feelings as well.

In most cases there are actions you can take to feel in control again. For instance, you can seek reassurance and understanding from others to make intense emotions less frightening. Body work such as exercise or yoga classes for pregnant women can make you feel more comfortable in your new body. Learning more about what awaits you in pregnancy and motherhood helps you accept changes in yourself. You can lessen your worries by making sure you are comfortable with your health care practitioner and informed about the medical routines. In pregnancy you thus amass an array of coping strategies, which will add to your competency as a mother.

Let me teach you about gratefulness. You have seen your Aunt Lisa. When your cousins whine, wanting dinner, a movie, and daddy right now, Lisa turns white, her jaw looks square, and her mouth shrinks to a pencil-thin line. You think she will commit murder, but instead she yells at her children to leave her alone and sends them to their rooms. After all she is bigger than they are and smarter, too.

Don't worry. I will not treat you this way. I will not lose my temper. I will understand. It is every child's right to whine. And to get sick, to pee in his pants, to spill on the carpet, and to tear mom's unread mail to shreds. Mother will make it all right again. It is what mothers are for. A mother will meet all the demands.

Oh, the demands on mothers! How can your cousins not see their mother's tired eyes?

You, my baby, are not even born yet. I have hemorrhoids and varicose veins. There is protein in my urine. Those huge vitamin pills get stuck in my throat. I cannot ride my bike anymore. You think it is no big deal, but it is to me. It is my freedom you are using as nourishment. You are so tiny and helpless and not even born yet, but you are already commanding me. I do not like the intrusion. I want my independence back. Leave me alone!

One of the most difficult emotions in pregnancy, which you will encounter again in motherhood, is resentment of your child. You thought you wanted this child so much, and now you find yourself resenting it. Such thoughts are frightening but common. Ambivalence is to be expected no matter how you longed for the child. There are many good reasons for this ambivalence. Facing the adjustments you will have to make in your life and realizing all the hard work involved are certainly not altogether pleasant.

There are other explanations for the emotionality of early motherhood, which take us into the deepest realms of our souls. The most significant is the bond between mother and child. It tests our capacities to form and support the most intimate and intense attachment we can have as adults. By nature this relationship evokes our most ardent and unadorned feelings. A child awakens memories and feelings from our own earliest experiences of being cared for. The reawakening of these emotions is good, because it enables us to identify with the child and understand what it is like to be so utterly dependent and vulnerable. At the same time, some of these emotions can be very painful. The extreme neediness of the child stirs up our own deepest hunger for maternal love and care. Some of us will be reminded of how devastating it was to be denied what we needed as children and of our inability to satisfy the infantile needs we carry with us as adults. When our own neediness is strong, there is always the frightening possibility that we will not be able to provide for a child in spite of our sincerest wishes to do so. When these feelings threaten us, we may respond with rage, disgust, and panic.

We have so much invested in our children. We want to give them the best, to make sure they get as good a start in life as we had ourselves, or perhaps a much better one. Yet at a subliminal level, we all have impossible expectations of what a son or daughter can give in return, whether it be someone who will admire and love us unconditionally, who will be a reflection of ourselves and a proof of our abilities, who can save a faltering marriage, or who can make us eternally happy and worry-free. We have dreams, hopes, expectations, and they all have very little to do with the real task of mothering a child. It is hard to admit these irrational and narcissistic wishes, and even harder to deal with the deep feelings that accompany them.

Conflictual emotions also arise in relation to a woman's inner self. Letting go of your old view of who you are and accepting who you are becoming are slow emotional processes, which contain all the elements of the loss of a loved one. For a time the new mother may not feel sure of who she is. The early relationship with the newborn requires her to be so open and attuned to the infant's needs that her own self blurs in with his as they temporarily exist as an undifferentiated twosome. In this state, she will find it difficult to get a clear grip on who she is. The new mother feels lost, even obliterated. Is it so strange that she is silently resentful of the child who intrudes upon her innermost self?

What kind of mother will I be when I cannot even get through pregnancy without whining? I am carrying you my child, so tender and pure, and I am poisoning you with my ill temper. I am drizzling my wicked brew onto your translucent skin, and naked you receive it. Wicked, wicked power of a woman embracing her child in the womb!

I promise I will change. Wait until I can hold your innocence in my arms. I will treasure you every moment. I will kiss your smooth forehead and tiny little fingers. I will whisper in your ear with a golden voice. You will know that my love is true and you will forgive me.

Guilt, the feeling many of us see as perennially associated with mothers, often follows resentment. Few admit having negative feelings toward their children. Such feelings are far from the serene love mothers "should" be feeling, and out of fear of being thought bad mothers, women do not like to talk about them. Thus, we are all left on our own to handle these difficult emotions.

Guilt creeps in when you think you do not measure up to the notion of what a good mother should be. And, yes, it is possible to feel blameworthy even before your child is born: Shouldn't you spend more time dreaming about your baby? Isn't it terribly selfish to choose to do things for your own pleasure instead? And how come you do not know as much about infants as the other women in your childbirth class? There is, no doubt, a lesson to be learned about motherhood even at this early stage. Pregnancy offers practice in distinguishing between uncalled-for guilt and that which you have rightfully earned.

Guilt, resentment, anxiety—these feelings hardly make pregnancy fun. Yet, along with all the other emotions they are at the heart of what makes you ready for the task of mothering. An honest exploration of them gives you a clearer understanding of who you are becoming. They help you find that inner source of strength that says that you are ready to accept your child.

USING INTUITION IN MOTHERHOOD

It was the cat that diverted Anna'a attention from Project Baby. Anna first saw her walking in proud, undaunted strides across the hardwood floor of her livingroom. The cat's gray-streaked fur, shabby and tangled, barely covered the lean body. You could see the long row of ribs sway from side to side as she moved. The cat had four kittens. She carried them in her mouth one by one. Gracefully she leaped up onto the old chest in the bay window. Anna was afraid the cat would drop her kittens as they dangled from her mouth, but the cat held on securely.

The cat chose a spot where the late afternoon sun hit the shiny oak surface. She shook her sleek body and the kittens dropped down one by one, dust and hairs dancing around them.

"You are cruel!" Anna gasped, but the cat did not pay any attention. She lay down, resting her head on her paws, and soon her rhythmic purr sang out lustfully. The kittens quickly crawled up against her middle and started sucking on her nipples. One of them lost his way. He was quickly whisked up by his mother's paw the moment his back legs dropped over the edge of the chest.

"Why are you here?" Anna asked. "Why do you hang around me? What do you want?"

The cat did not move. Anna saw her contentment. This animal did not need anything from her. No, it was the other way around. The cat was there for Anna's sake. In her silent, canny manner she was there to teach Anna.

But what could this ragged-looking cat, who almost seemed to ignore her four furry kitten-balls, teach her? The cat knew nothing about a pregnant human's worries, what it was like to have a mind that asked how, how, how, when she thought about herself with a child.

"What is your secret, cat?" Anna asked. "How can you be so confident? How do you know how to mother?"

A renewed connection with your intuitive side often takes place in pregnancy. Together with your feelings intuition can be pivotal in helping you build a solid sense of yourself as a mother. Many women claim to feel more intuitive while carrying their children, as if the felt-but not-seen child connects them to this inner strength. Thus they may "sense" the sex of the baby, "know" what to eat or what activities to avoid, "feel" when something is not quite right with the baby or when delivery is imminent—all without having any convincing arguments to back up their claims. If nurtured, this heightened sensitivity will continue into motherhood.

Sometimes using your intuition as a parent means trusting your first impulse. A parent may sense there is something wrong with his or her child before there are any overt signs to confirm it. Or, although no dictionary can help with the interpretation, you can learn to discriminate between the different cries of an infant. At other times you need patience to let a decision slowly grow from within. This may mean waiting until you feel it is the right moment to wean or to leave your child in someone else's care.

Belief in one's intuitive powers is often frowned upon. Regarded as irrational, subjective, nebulous, and vague, intuition is dismissed as a way to mother skillfully. Undoubtedly, it is foolish to think that something so overromanticized and difficult to define as the "mother instinct" can always guide us to act appropriately toward our children. Yet, ultimately we must learn to trust our intuition of what is best for the child. Intuition is necessary in many situations where there is no absolute right or wrong or we simply have not been taught what to do. Motherhood cannot be merely a product of our rational minds. It must also be founded in our very personal feelings and our intuitive sense—both of which allow us to build the strong and flexible selves that are essential in caring for a child.

The knowledge you acquire by listening inward is different from the knowledge you get from the authorities on child care. It is highly personal and based on your uniqueness. No one can tell you what is right or wrong. From it comes the independence you need to be able to take your stand against all the contrary advice you receive, whether it comes from professionals or friends. Your own views can be much more valuable than the opinions of others. After all, your unique way of using your power and authority is the most important factor in your child's well-being.

Cat in the bay window. I think I am starting to understand why you hang around me. You do not scare me anymore. I no longer think you will hurt your kittens. Now I can see that you cannot help but take care of them. In your animal veins flows a stream that urges you to care and protect. What does it matter that you are so scrubby and bony, that you seem to carry your kittens carelessly, that you live free and independent and lie idle in the sun? Your kittens are not concerned. They trust.

I, too, am starting to trust. I will listen to the humming stream of life inside myself and know that I, too, have mother-blood.

If you let your feelings and intuition guide you into motherhood you will learn to trust yourself. When you believe in the goodness of your unique way of caring for your child, you have truly accepted yourself as a mother. Stepping away from the professional attitude, so easy to adopt when you are unsure of yourself, will give the confidence you can have only when motherhood is rooted inside.

Chapter 2

THE PERFECT MOTHER

"Take a good look at my mother manual. I have constructed it with utmost care. I have picked out all the facts and figures needed to ensure I give good care. These guidelines are my guarantee that hasty judgment will not trick me. I am opting for my child's best, there will not be one mistake.

Nursing, bathing, and navel care: how I hope I know it all. May my touch be light and gentle and convey the feelings I hold inside. Honesty will be my watchword, always showing what I truly feel. Happy, stable, manners mild, for outbursts can confuse a child.

The planning stage will soon be over. Now all details must connect. I will add the final entries and just hope the manual for mothering is correct."

"No." Anna shrugs off her thoughts as if they were a swarm of summer flies feasting on a horse's hide. "Of course not. There are no mothering manuals in real life." She knows that. Yet, how she wishes motherhood could be premeditated. She wants Miriam to trust that mother knows what she is doing.

As we in pregnancy try to imagine what it will be like to have a child, we gather a collection of expectations and ideals that stay with us into motherhood. Some of these expectations date back to our own childhood, others are created in pregnancy as we envision ourselves as mothers, and many are adopted from society's images of the ideal mother. By the time the child is born, the mothering manual has grown into a heavy volume of guidelines for parental success that will inspire as well as intimidate.

For many of us it is not enough to become what child psychiatrist D. W. Winnicott called "a good enough mother," a mother who trusts that her common sense will guide her in caring for her child. Our genuine efforts are transformed into a compulsive preoccupation with always working toward our own excellence, a task that is, as we shall see, as cumbersome as it is futile.

The compulsive need to be perfect sneaks into the picture in pregnancy when the pregnant women is determined to get everything just right: Has she chosen the right diet, exercise program, physician, and maternity class? Does she have the best possible stroller, infant seat, pacifier, and receiving blanket? Is her pregnant body under her control, not over the average weight gain for the trimester, no cellulites or loose skin hiding under her clothes, and how is the blood count this week? Has the child growing in utero had his daily dose of rhythms and music, small talk from daddy, oxygen-rich blood from his mother's workout? Modern mothering ideals even propose a perfect way to deliver a baby: usually a drug-free, vaginal delivery facilitated by husband, soothing music, and positive affirmations.

After the child is born, the drive for perfection continues in the heavy investment the new parents make in caring for their newborn. The child must be ensured his share of educational toys, infant swim and parent-child creativity hours, early enrollment in the best academic classes, and of course high-quality time with mom and dad. Baby's behavioral progress is carefully monitored and labeled according to some external measure of success: the first smile came right on schedule, he was a bit late with his first teeth but luckily he crawled early, and so on. The child's progress is the measure of how well the parents are doing.

The pursuit of perfection is an illusion that has us convinced that we will be good parents if and when we can do it just right. If only we set our minds to it and become more loving, tolerant, organized, or educated—to name a few desired qualities—we can finally relax and enjoy parenthood. Regrettably, we always seem to fall short. Then we feel guilty for our wrongdoing, and hate ourselves, too, for not getting it right this time, either. Ah, the marvels of parenthood—what is wrong with us that we cannot quite seem to achieve it? The experience of motherhood is instead infested with feelings of guilt and self-reproach.

The self-confidence of your typical new parent is more than shaky, it is overhauled. Sadly, it is as if our generation does not trust that we in ourselves are enough for our children. We feel that we must back up our presence in our children's lives with the "right" activities, preferably endorsed by experts, and watch carefully for any sign that we, after all, are doing something wrong.

Like their parents, children are also negatively affected by their parent's perfectionism. "Our intensity about parenting, heightened by the overwhelming amount of advice available to us, has placed us in the precarious position of creating 'too precious' children," says Sally James.[1] When parents try too hard, for instance, by showering their children with attention, incessantly manipulating their environment, or doing everything to prevent conflicts, the children learn that there are a right and a wrong way to be a child, she argues. The children do not learn how to trust themselves to do what is right. Nor do they learn that the world is not and does not have to be perfect, and that in fact there are lessons to be learned from your failures.

The appreciation of pregnancy as a transformative experience in our lives, a wonderous moment in life to be savored and taken into the bloodstream of our souls, is lost when we are trapped in the throes of perfectionism. Marion Woodman says, "To move towards perfectionism is to move out of life, or what is worse, never to enter it."[2] Perfectionism and intellectualization (as in *Project Baby*) are sisters in the same peapod. All our mental and spiritual energy goes into the pursuit of these ideas, and nothing is left to nourish our inner transformations to mothers. We work so hard to achieve what in reality is impossible, and in the process the appreciation of the wonders of pregnancy and birth, all the hard work we put into this creative act, and our ability to appreciate our children slip out of our hands.

THE PREGNANT WOMAN: EXPECTATIONS RUNNING HIGH

My child, at four months you are only a bundle of fetal tissue, cartilage, and cell layers the size of my closed fist. What life will be yours? I do not know. The blueprint of your future is contained within the memory of each cell. Like studying the pattern of leaves in a teacup I wish I could look for answers in your intricate strands of DNA.

I never learned how to do a full split. My hamstrings were too tight. And my fingers were not long enough to reach between low C and high E on the keyboard. Perhaps one day I will see you surpass me. You could teach me about organic solvents, laboratory reagents, and the molecular weight of phosphoric acid. You might mention your past in the foreword to your first photographic portfolio. You could be reciting Milton to an audience of tired teenagers. I will be watching you try out your wings from the back porch, reminiscing about the day, not long ago, when you were nothing but a bundle of nerve-endings connecting with tissue deep inside my body.

As long as you are carrying the child in the womb it can be anything you want it to be: boy or girl, curly dark charmer or fair blonde, the Picasso, Madonna, or Albert Einstein of the future—the possibilities are endless. The child will assume the identity you always wanted; in fact, it will assume all ninety of them. There are no limits for the child who has not yet made any blunders in life. Your child can take your own achievements one step further, and with your assistance he will not have to make any foolish mistakes. The road to success is already at his feet, and all he has to do is to follow your directions.

Your child's infancy is also painted by imagination's sweet intemperance. How do you picture you and your baby together? Is your little pumpkin perhaps always happy and smiling; never cross, crying, or colicky; and if by any chance he is a little bit out of it, will you not immediately know how to restore him to a blissful state again? Other children may be cranky and obnoxious, but such nuisances are due to their parent's ignorance. Your own method is significantly improved, thanks to other parents' striking demonstration of what not to do. Your treasured time with your sweetheart will be spent filling your lungs with pure and fresh baby-smell, brushing the fluffy hair on her head, powdering her soft bottom, and skillfully applying a knob of ointment, then lovingly rocking her to sleep. But most importantly you will get to know each other, you will entice her toothless smiles, babble, and make funny faces together. Ah, this is what motherhood is all about and you want it NOW!

In pregnancy we can dream undisturbed both about our children and about ourselves as mothers. The excitement and love we already feel toward the unborn child color our vision of ourselves as parents. We assume that our willingness to give of ourselves is strong enough to eliminate our shortcomings and to bring out the wisdom we will need to mother well.

The dreams in pretty pink and blue that we dream in pregnancy are colored, among other things, by our motivations for having a child. If we are willing to examine our fantasies, we will most likely find some interesting notions of what we expect to get from the experience. Angela Barron-McBride says bluntly in *The Growth and Development of Mothers*: "How many have babies simply and solely 'because they love children'? Very few indeed, I suspect. Even when children are wanted and planned for (something that is not as common as one might think, even among those who are sophisticated about birth control), people have babies for reasons that have nothing to do with loving children."[3] Behind the wish for a child we can find a long list of secret requests for rewards and gratifications that upon examination prove embarrassingly irrational. Some of us hope that a child can provide us with a life change of such potency that it will blow away our present troubles. Others think that having a child will ward off our low self-esteem; make us feel needed, younger, livelier, and happier; or give us a chance to show our adult maturity. We may want to please our parents by making them grandparents. Yet others wish that a child will improve a halting marriage. Surely motherhood will boost our self-esteem through our parental endeavors and through the admiring look we will see in our children's eyes. Thus we hope that becoming a mother will bestow on us whatever qualities or circumstances we think we are lacking.

As new mothers, we have the necessary but difficult task of renegotiating these inner directives so they better fit reality and of coming to terms with the discrepancies among what kind of mother you want your child to have, what kind of child you want as a mother, and what it turns out that the two of you actually get. Although it certainly provokes concern when you become aware of how self-serving your motivations for having a child may be, remember that most of them will wear off after the child is born. In any case, it is not possible to do away with them prematurely. In the course of time, as you and your child get to know each other, preconceptions will be replaced by relationship and you will come to appreciate your child for what he or she is.

GOOD MOTHERS AND PERFECT MOTHERS

Sometimes it is difficult to understand the difference between our efforts to be good mothers and our wishes to be perfect mothers. The difference is in how we treat the mistakes we inevitably will make as new mothers. A woman can normally keep her self-esteem reasonably intact even when she faces difficulties. She is confident that she will be able to cope with most situations. She soon recovers from her mistakes and becomes a good deal wiser, too. If she, on the other hand, is besieged by perfectionism, her tendency to self-reproach will govern her actions. She simply cannot allow herself to do anything that would feed her low self-worth. Instead of expecting to learn from her mistakes, she so fears the consequences that she will map out her every action in an attempt to avoid the mistakes before they happen.

The motivations for the wish to become a good mother and the wish to be perfect are the same: As a mother you want what is best for your child. *Your child deserves that the most important woman in his life gives her best effort to care for him.* To be able to give generously and benevolently of yourself is both an exciting and a rewarding part of the mothering experience. Every mother issues severe prescriptions for herself out of love for her child. We can imagine this sense of responsibility be a natural part of motherhood that can be traced back through the generations like the annual rings of a tree trunk. The force of love is indeed magically powerful, urging us to do anything possible to ensure that our children can feel our love.

Even our best intentions can work against us. What, for example, happens when the wish to do a good job grows so out of proportion that our mother ideal no longer is a glistening star inspiring us to new heights but a dense fog in which we cannot navigate? What happens when our expectations turn into inner commands that rule our every thought and action with iron-fast determination? And what happens to our abilities to mother when the desire to be the best parent possible turns into an obsession? Let us see what we can learn about the hazards of our transformation to mothers from the following dismal portrayal of the worst-case perfectionist.

PORTRAIT OF THE PERFECT MOTHER

I cannot do this. It is too difficult. My daughter, is it possible that I have failed you long before you lie warm and wet on my stomach?

Like a false labor contraction squeezing my uterus tight, closing in on my child and the constricted space she occupies within me, my worries trap me inside.

There is a way out; there must be. One that I have yet overlooked. I must return to my mission. Try a little harder; try again.

If we hold our breath through the tightening, long enough for the fresh air to plummet down in a gush of new hope, then we are free again.

Please follow the list and do not diverge again:
One receiving blanket in color of your choice
Four to six diaper covers
Cotton underwear with snaps in the crotch
Three or more one-piece outfits
A bassinet with flannel sheets, sheepskin optional.

The unfortunate woman who is caught in the sticky web of perfectionism faces the same task in pregnancy that all mothers do—she is searching for the best imaginable way to mother her child. Yet, for this woman the search becomes an exhausting preoccupation. Every detail concerning her child must be planned, every alternative explored. Nothing can be left to chance or improvisation, since the lack of reflection this indicates does not ensure that the perfect choice will be made. To be caught ignorant and uninformed in a subject would be to let loose the anguished doubts she carries inside.

The watchful stance may be quite exhausting, but it is the only way she can stay in perfect control and not be caught off guard. How else could she be ready to embark upon every new subject she encounters and to find satisfying answers for those gnawing questions inside: Am I doing the right thing? Am I sure this is the very best alternative? Are there any facts and figures that I have overlooked? What else is there to know?

The devotion to perfectionism makes a woman intolerant and judgmental. She is governed by a merciless voice that dictates and rejects any behavior or emotion that is not quite perfect. Slowly, the ability to overlook and forgive is lost. What is left are the hardening lumps of what she should do and what she must do: As a mother, she must always be fair and consistent, she should be home during the child 's first year, she has to stop being so selfish, she must never lose patience with her child, or whatever else her personal orders dictate. She must follow the commands to the letter or meet an unthinkable, horrible fate: To become a mother whose blemished character will destroy the innocent child left in her care.

The voice that lives within the perfectionist is dreadfully tyrannical, yet it is not likely that the woman questions its existence. She is too used to her tormentor to believe that the situation can be different. The demands the woman puts on herself as a mother did not emerge along with her pregnancy; they are a part of the wickerwork of her feminine psyche. Before her pregnancy the perfectionistic attitude may have concerned her appearance, or her performance as an employee, lover, friend, or daughter. All moves had to be perfect or she would fall into an emotional muddle of galling worthlessness. Yet, in motherhood the demands will be even more ruthless. Suddenly the stakes are much higher. Now her anxiety concerns not only her own self but how she will succeed with someone she feels so much love and compassion for—her own child.

There is no room for closeness in perfectionism. The perfectionist fears the self-loathing and shame that would overwhelm her if someone revealed the flaws she cannot even acknowledge to herself. Solitude and isolation threaten to be her sole companions in motherhood. Perhaps she does not believe that other women can be of any help to her. Motherhood is a struggle she must conquer alone. Consequently, she misses out on the opportunity to learn in the company of other young mothers that mistakes can be made, laughed at, and forgiven.

What is it like to be in the presence of the Perfect Mother? As you listen to her convincing words about motherhood it becomes obvious that she is right and your own ideas so trivial and inadequate. Maybe there is a sudden yearning to be like her, so confident and right. But how could you possibly measure up? You shrink into feelings of inferiority like plastic-wrap scorched on the hot stove. In your own interest, you will then shy away, knowing that you cannot beat her at her game. She is too good at proving her point with bullet-proof reasoning. If you stay around, you will be stuck in negative feelings. Likewise, the contempt she implies for any form of weakness is an efficient weapon. Her message is clear both on an intellectual and on an emotional frequency: Stay away!

Is the perfect mother within you? Is she ready to take over when you become a mother? From the intellectual distance that *reading* about perfectionism allows we can all ascertain that we will not engage in such self-destructive activities as parents. We can safely admit to and laugh at our own personal version of the desire for perfection. Yet, when reality removes us from the point of observation we may well react differently. In the midst of an activity so completely new and important to us as mothering, feelings of inadequacy can surprise our reasoning minds. When the cries of the newborn pierce the new parent like daggers and she fails to calm the baby down, few will convincingly argue that they are not at fault. Liberal doses of compassion not only for the baby but for ourselves are called for, yet often difficult to summon.

How did we lose confidence that we would become good mothers naturally? Why are we so hard on ourselves as mothers? When did our critical minds take over to dictate what motherhood should be like? To find answers we will turn our attention away from the personal portrait and look for clues beyond our immediate surroundings.

THE CULTURAL IDEALIZATION OF MOTHERS

Sylvia, Anna's supervisor, how does she do it? Three spirited children, ages seven, four, and two, who fill her house with play and laughter. There is always a family crisis to cope with: Chicken pox and ear infections, the baby-sitter is leaving and must be replaced before the end of the month, and Evan has his arm in a cast. Lynn throws horrible temper tantrums, Seth does not like his preschool, and where will she find money for Evan's emergency dental care?

Sylvia, family manager. Always busy, always in demand. She keeps the activities running smoothly and finds creative solutions to every practical dilemma. Sylvia is the flywheel that keeps her bustling family in balance.

Does Sylvia ever reflect on what she is doing? Does she ever question her way of mothering? Anna doubts she does. Sylvia just knows what to do. She does not dwell on how other parents handle their children.

Anna is light-years away from assuming Sylvia's motherly presence. She observes, attentively, from her place at the edge of Sylvia's family life. Perhaps she will get a taste of what motherliness feels like. What does the pride of seeing your children thrive feel like? Will it matter to have so little time to yourself? What does it feel like to be so utterly needed?

Anna must watch and absorb as much as she can. Soon it will be her turn.

The cultural idealization of motherhood is an important reason behind perfectionism. As insecure mothers-to-be and new mothers we are particularly sensitive to suggestions of how we should behave as mothers. Society's idea of the perfect mother is presented to us through the lens of the exaggeration-prone media and in the advice our child care experts provide us with. Their representations of motherhood have one thing in common: They imply that these ideals both *are* achievable and *should* be achieved by every mother. If we take motherhood seriously, we must be careful not to embarrass ourselves by bleak comparisons to the stereotype.

What characterizes the ideal mother whom we would gladly sell our hair to be like? Although noble qualities vary from individual to individual, we can still easily find some common denominators among us. For the modern woman of the nineties, the ideal mother, is something like this: She is loving, caring, comforting, passionate, understanding, creative, enthusiastic, devoted, unselfish, conscientuous, and very educated and skillful in child care matters. She is never domineering, selfish, depressed, bored, hot-tempered, scheming, impatient, unempathic, tired, or bitchy. Not only is she perfect when she is with her children, she also manages to be a sexy wife and an interesting partner; a successful, assertive, independent, aggressive, creative, wealthy career woman; and a whiz at self-actualization. Some of these values have been tagged onto the mother role for generations; others are a function of recent changes in the ideals associated with womanhood.

In the early and mid-1900s, serving the needs of others was considered natural to a woman's character. There was never any question of conflict between a woman's needs as an individual and her role as a caregiver. Today, we have one set of values for what women should be like as active members of society and another for what they must do to be good mothers, and these two are often in collision.[4] For example, you cannot simultaneously "be there" for your child and make sure the bills are paid and your career advancing. Every woman must set her priorities and make her choices and then live with the consequences, usually feelings of frustration and guilt when her commitments suffer.

Our new ideals of womanhood have intensified the guilt feelings long since associated with motherhood. Women used to feel guilty when they failed to enjoy motherhood and produce the perfect children the way society expected them to do. These expectations have hardly disappeared from the mother role. We still consider ourselves responsible for our children's behavior. Yet, nowadays the guilt feelings not only concern our performance as mothers but are the price we pay for our new freedom of choice and the inevitable conflict of interests that follows. If your time is divided between mothering and meeting other responsibilities, you had better make up for your absences by being an extremely good mother when you are with your child. Furthermore, if you have voluntarily chosen pregnancy and know that the number of children you will have is limited (the national average is 1.9 children per woman),[5] you are determined to get it right the first time. Under these circumstances, perfectionism can thrive.

Perfectionism is not exclusive to women. Men, too, can become preoccupied with their performance as fathers. The stereotype of a good father depicts a man who is the provider and protector of the family. Nowadays we also encourage his direct involvement with his children. The new father is caught in the conflict between what is expected from him publicly and at home, and he is pressured to perform well in both areas. In his favor is the plain fact that he does not have the weight of traditional role patterns that assumes his succesfulness as a caregiver. A man's involvement with his children is considered new and exciting, whereas a woman's participation is more or less taken for granted. He can thus afford to err, while her confusion may be pronounced a risk to her child's development.

THE SCIENTIFICALLY CONTROLLED PREGNANCY

There are three pregnant women at Winston & Garvey this year: Beatrice, soon full-term and still stunningly attractive in her tailored maternity suits; Rianne, her stomach protruding farther out than Beatrice's even though she is six weeks behind her; and Anna, who looks girlishly slender in comparison to the other two. The three of them seek each other out to chat about the topic they all prioritize. As Anna passes the copy room on her way to the bathroom, she sees Beatrice and Rianne leaning their tired backs against the Fax machine. Anna can tell by the intensity of their conversation that they are discussing baby matters.

"I think it is important to be in a familiar environment. I will feel much calmer if I can surround myself with my usual mess at home."

"I would never dare to give birth at home. I want all the medical attention I can get. To be honest with you, I am hoping for a Cesarean. How nice it would be to avoid the pain of a vaginal delivery."

"You can't be serious! Think about your poor child. What a shock to him to be cut out of your womb in a few quick minutes."

"I don't think he is capable of telling the difference, dear."

"You never know. Infants are incredibly alert after natural births. Why would you want to cloud your very first meeting in drowsiness? I would personally like to greet my son with all senses open, and at home, where he belongs."

"I want a memorable birth as well, but why must the experience be painful, and why take the risks of a home delivery?"

"If you would rather not have a natural delivery, I assume that you will not want to breastfeed either?"

"Sure, I do. It is the best way to form a secure relationship with your child."

"Absolutely. And how nice to know that your child gets adequate nutrition and protection from your immune system."

The two women turn to Anna in a moment of silence. Anna clears her throat.

"I haven't quite made up my mind yet," she says apologetically.

"Oh, you do right to take your time. It is important to take in the facts first."

"Yes, there is so much to make up one's mind about. No wonder we waited so long to have children."

"It is the reason we are so neurotic about having them."

Anna makes a simple excuse and leaves the other two to their conversation. In the competition of who is the most knowledgeable of the three, Anna is clearly the loser. Motherhood is a task the other two already seem to be on their way to mastering. Where do they hide the wretched uncertainty that lives in Anna?

Our society encourages us to improve and perfect our performances continuously. We are valued for what we do and how well we do it. We are expected to look for excellence, whether it be in the president with the perfect record, the athlete with no losses, or the student with straight A's. Their excellence becomes our personal measure of success, and when our humanness inevitably shines through we are seriously disillusioned.

Parents, and mothers in particular, are subject to the same cultural idealization and subsequent fall from grace. The old saying "the hand that rocks the cradle is the hand that rules the nation" demonstrates how seriously we take our parental duties. Our parenting efforts are of national importance and should not to be taken lightly. Parents are responsible for raising good citizens, and ever since Rousseau, mothers have been considered naturally suited to this task.[6] Society readily dictates what mothers should do to produce exceptional children, yet in the end mothers alone are presumably responsible for the outcome.

Motherhood is judged against the same competitive standard as our other enterprises in society. As we begin to adapt to the new and challenging role of parenting it feels right and safe to rely on well-known measures of success. We judge our efforts according to how productive, efficient, and clever we are, as measured by our children's progress. Did we manage to give birth to an alert newborn? Is the baby nursing appropriately? Is he developing faster, or at least *en par* with the norm? Questions concerning diet, health, daily routines, and early education often cause a fervid preoccupation that goes far above any real interest in the matters. The need to control every little detail has less to do with what is necessary to protect the child than with attempts to prove that we will be good mothers.

Modern pregnancy care has accustomed us to viewing pregnancy as a medical condition that to a great degree can be manipulated. There are blood and urine tests, ultrasound examinations, and fetal monitors to ensure that gestation follows a normal course. If problems arise there are many surgical and medical procedures that can restore the health of both mother and child.

It may be forgiven us if we assume that we should be able to control our psychological transformation to mothers as well. If instrumental reasoning determines how we perceive ourselves as mothers-to-be, we will assume that it is our duty to control as much as possible of the process of becoming a mother. We deceive ourselves to believe that almost anything can be controlled in pregnancy, that if only we do x, y, and z the child of our dreams, a child whose future we have the power to shape into whatever we consider to be for his or her own good, will be born.

That we are led astray may seem incomprehensible when there are professionals to turn to for questions about our children. But how much help can these services be if the sense of being lost comes from within, when we have difficulties perceiving ourselves as competent mothers? It is sad to see how so many of us lack the inner confidence that can reassure as well as encourage to find help when needed. Instead we turn to authorities who are child care experts yet who often know little about what women need to be nurturing mothers.

In the negative sense, to control your performance as a parent means that you will rely exclusively on outer dictates to make your decisions. It is the need always to think strategically, to have a master plan for all of your interactions with your child, to cover every conceivable risk, and to demand measurable results of yourself. It is to give no authority to your intuition and never let your feelings or heart guide you. This stern attitude fits well into the strategy we have focused on as women of the nineties: the rational, goal-oriented strategy side of ourselves that will embrace yet another field in which to be ambitious and competitive. We let the standards that guide us professionally apply to the mother role as well.

Our tireless pursuit of perfection sabotages our attempts to look at the powers we as individuals already have in our possession. It leads us away from the task of building inner confidence. This confidence comes forth when our personal resources are honored and seen as crucial to the process of becoming a mother. We must take time to go over our personal assets and envision how these may help us to mother. Only when we can believe in the worth of our own opinions and conclusions can we set other standards for motherhood than what society presently suggests. If we as mothers accept responsibility for our children's well-being, we should do so not because we feel pressured by a society that likes to hold mothers accountable, but because we have deliberately chosen *how* we mother and thus will accept responsibility for the decisions we have made.

THE PERFECT MOTHER AND HER PAST

In addition to the pressure society puts on us as parents, some of us are lugging around some heavy emotional baggage from our past that makes us extra vulnerable to becoming perfection-seeking mothers. Many of us have never learned to accept and love ourselves fully. We therefore look to the outside for approval in an effort to compensate for our inferiority feelings. These narcissistic wounds of our past become extra sensitized when we take on motherhood.

"The attempt to be an ideal parent, that is to behave correctly toward the child, to raise her correctly, not to give too little or too much, is in essence an attempt to be the ideal child—well behaved and dutiful—of one's own parents,"[7] says Alice Miller. The famous Swiss psychoanalyst represents the theorists who find the reason for compulsive behaviors and constant low self-esteem in our childhood. The eternal hope that this time you, the beloved child of your parents, will finally do something right creeps into your adult dreams about becoming a mother. In your dreams, motherhood will be the ultimate test of your own worth.

The injustice done to you as a child, of never having been loved for who you are, may now shadow your relationship with your child. It is difficult to listen to your child with empathy and understanding if you are preoccupied with being a good mother. In striving to meet your expectations of what the ideal mother-child relationship should be like, the emotional needs of your child may go unnoticed. The child in turn learns to hide his or her true feelings and to do whatever is necessary to please mother. He is taught that there are a right and a wrong way to be a child.

Alice Miller uses the phrase "the Poisonous Pedagogy" to describe the child-rearing methods she considers to be damaging to children. She criticizes these systematic attempts to procure obedience and control for producing emotionally crippled children. The discipline designed to be "for the children's own good" is in reality an unconscious attempt to meet the needs of the adult. When their parents do not validate the emotions that express who they are, children become afraid and ashamed of their feelings. They begin to hide and suppress their emotions until intellect and emotions no longer are connected in their self-awareness. The development of a healthy sense of self is severed.

Dr. Miller's message is clear and sobering: A parent's neurotic need to direct parenthood according to his own childhood script will lead to the destruction of the child's free spirit. As parents we are, indeed, responsible for the psychological well-being of the next generation.

When it is time for motherhood, the woman who carries emotional wounds from her past will try to become the perfect mother as a way to make up for her own unhappy childhood. This is her chance to create the happy childhood she never had herself, and to be the mother she never had herself. She hopes that her child will not suffer as she once did. But the unhealed scars from her past get in the way. Instead of helping her child's life to unfold and take its own course, she unwittingly tries to conduct her child's life in such a way that she will get her own needs met. She will also tie her own self-worth to her child's conduct. When her child behaves well, she feels proud of her achievement as a parent, and when the child misbehaves, she sees it as a sign of her own failure.

"Many women are still trying to achieve self-definition through a performance aimed at pleasing and being accepted,"[8] says Colette Dowling in her book *Perfect Women*. In whatever activity we engage in as women, we work until we drop to achieve recognition and admiration for our deeds. Dowling points out how ironic it is that the possibilities that have opened up to women during the last decades have supported the illusion that we will feel terrific if only we do enough and do it well enough. Yet, in spite of our new powers in society many women still feel weak and inferior inside, something we try to hide with even more achievements.

"The drive to become better is a compulsion, a never-ending quest for admiration because there's nothing warming us from within,"[9] Dowling says. Since the woman who has learned to disparage herself is prevented from developing a "true self," she becomes dependent on others to fill her inner emptiness. The origin of the inner harshness that characterizes the narcissistically wounded woman can be found in the early mother-daughter relationship. Mother is the person who provides us with the first and most important inner representation of ourselves. Colette Dowling's view agrees with that of Alice Miller: If a child's mother thinks little of herself, she will look to her daughter to provide her with self-worth. She will communicate to her daughter that she is responsible for her mother's happiness. The daughter must hide her true feelings in order to be loved. As an adult she will continue to look for others' acceptance in order to feel self-worth, just as her mother once tried to redeem herself through her daughter.

Passing on emotional legacies is not something that only people who have been severely neglected as children tend to do. We are all tarnished products of our less-than perfect upbringings. No one has had the Perfect Childhood. We have internalized the emotional and behavioral patterns of our families of origin, and these in turn shape how we perceive ourselves, the world, and our relationships as adults. With our children we tend to recreate the themes of our unresolved past.

This deterministic view of our psychological lives is far from consoling to the parent-to-be. And thanks to the popularization of psychodevelopmental theories, most of us carry around some version of *Why My Childhood Made Me to Who I Am* that comes in handy to explain our adult misfortunes and incorrigible behaviors. Yet, it would be a mistake to conclude that our childhood scars inescapably repeat themselves in our children. Awareness of our emotional traumas is also a prerequisite for change. We must remember that we will find the healthy desire to resolve our childhood traumas beneath the compulsion to recreate the situations that led to our psychological difficulties. When we can be forgiving and compassionate with ourselves and win the courage to look into our destructive powers as parents, we can use our insight to look for more appropriate behaviors. Breaking our habitual responses is, however, not an easy task. Enlightenment requires hard, ongoing work and much practice and often the gracious support of a good *role mother*.[10]

IMPERFECT MOTHERING

How do you as a parent encourage a healthy sense of self in your child if perfectionism tends to get in your way? Developmental psychology identifies three important stages in a child's emotional development in which you as a parent play a crucial role. These are the stages of bonding, mirroring, and separation-individuation.[11] The first stage, bonding, can be said to begin in pregnancy as you daydream about the child in utero. You feel warmth and love toward your expected child, hold little loving conversations with him, and delight in the first signs of life. The prebirth acquaintence is where you begin to build the psychological attachment to your child that will help you read and respond to his needs once your close physical bond is broken. When a child has a trusting and secure relationship to his parents, he develops the inner strength that will help him through the frustrations and disappointments of life without losing his sense of self. He also learns to form loving and intimate relationships. Thus, in pregnancy and motherhood alike, it is more important to give yourself time with your child than to be concerned that you are doing everything just right.

The second stage in a child's emotional development, mirroring, takes place when you as a parent help your child see himself as he truly is. You help him identify his own emotional experiences with your words, gestures, and affection. Paris and Paris describe mirroring as an act of love in which the parent tells his child,

> I'll be with you while you grow. I'll pay attention to what you tell me—with your words, with your body, and with your behavior. I will be present and will make every effort to understand your feelings and help you understand yourself. I will assist you with your difficulties without making you wrong. I'll make our relationship safe enough for you to risk expressing directly your authentic feelings.[12]

Finally, separation-individuation is the process in which a child learns to differentiate himself emotionally from his caretakers and develop his own thoughts and feelings—he learns that there are a Me and a You. Your role in this process is to convey to your child that he can have his separate thoughts and feelings without losing his connection with you. You will gradually let go of your involvement and accept your child's first steps toward independence.

Just as we find it important to support our children's intellectual development, we must learn to value and nourish their emotional development. Without a healthy sense of self, children's unique talents and interests cannot thrive. Sensitive and caring attention to their emotional needs is our primary task as new parents. As our children grow, we must find the means to identify when and how we transmit the dysfunctional behaviors we carry with us from our past to them. You may for example notice how you try to distract or discipline your child when he displays feelings you cannot tolerate in yourself. You may also discover that you are so set on creating the perfect child that you forget to leave room for your child's unique needs and interests. If you can extend yourself to love your child's ordinariness as well as his specialness, you will nurture a healthy sense of self in him and also take steps to learn a healthy attitude toward your own weaknesses. With good intentions and equally good advice, we can become mothers who create a sense of trust and safety in our children without hampering their development toward independence and self-reliance.

Parenting is an unglamorous learning process. Try to parent without the appreciation for the challenge and you set yourself up for failure. It takes a good deal of faith to trust that your first fumbling efforts are in fact a gold mine of good mothering. It may seem crazy to put your stakes on yourself when you look more like a halting mule than an elegant race-horse. Yet crazy you must be to trust that from inner scrubbiness and scantiness can emerge a mother as tough and spunky as an old mule. You may not look like much at first appearance, but bear with yourself and you will soon show your true potential.

THE MOTHER-SELF

Intellectual awareness of our typical beliefs and behaviors leads us away from the destructive patterns we otherwise might repeat with our children. Yet, one cannot mother on thoughts alone. At some point we need to leave the mind alone and go searching for the heart, in the realm of the warmth and feeling that feed the human spirit. Here we will find the keeper of the aliveness we want to radiate to our children. We can call this place the mother-self. The mother-self is a place inside that guides our interactions with our children. We can also turn here for comfort and support when parenthood overwhelms us. It is a place where the ego can rest and accomplishments and failures do not matter. Here we will find our true feelings about ourselves and our children, regardless of the stresses of the moment. From the mother-self mothering comes forth with passion.

Jack Lee Rosenberg and Marjorie Rand of the Institute of Integrative Body Psychotherapy in Venice, California, define *the sense of self* as "a non-verbal experience of well-being, identity, and continuity that is felt in the body."[13] They claim that we cannot separate our bodily experiences from our mental perceptions of who we are. The inner relationship we have to our selves is manifested in our bodily posture, voice, muscle tension, and movement patterns. A healthy sense of self develops in childhood when our physical and emotional needs are met in a loving and satisfying way. However, if we are not given a pattern of feeling good and comfortable in our bodies at an early age, our emotional responses and belief systems become fixed in the musculature and we are blocked from experiencing a sense of well-being. The strength of the mother-self is a direct function of our capacity to experience pleasure in our bodies. We can return to the sensations of our maternal bodies to counteract the critical mind.

To regard body and self as inseparable is particularly interesting in pregnancy when both the psychological and physiological changes are so prominent. If it is true that our psychological characteristics are connected to our physique, we can assume that the physical changes in pregnancy will affect the self, so that emotions and sensations we normally are not in touch with can surface. This may account for the prevalence of anxiety and emotional pain that makes pregnancy so stressful. Although it is an unpleasant task, we are presented with a chance to work through, or at least become aware of, some of the deeply buried material that may affect our parenting abilities. Pregnancy cleanses us so that we are free to meet the child with our true selves.

The growing child in the body gradually makes room for us to experience a new and deeper connection to our selves. Aside from the pain of reexperiencing past traumas, there is also hope for new feelings of well-being and self-love to emerge. Perhaps for the first time in adulthood, we can leave the mind, where most of our preparations for motherhood take place, and let our lower bodies become the focal point. As will be discussed in later chapters, the womb and its sexual energy, instinctual wisdom, and life bearing creativity can become our greatest source of mothering.

We are so busy trying to get through pregnancy with honors that we lose track of the significance of the experience. The texture, color, and feel of pregnancy are as important to the transformation to mother as its structure. There are songs to be chanted, drums to be drummed upon, dances to be performed, and tales to be heard. These thoroughly unscientific matters of pregnancy give meaning and delight to what we are going through. Pregnancy helps us come to our senses.

There is no perfect procedure or right formula to follow in motherhood. It is not how well you manage to adhere to your ideals that will sail you through the rough spots of parenting but how you manage to stay true to yourself and hang on to your love and respect for your child. If you can learn to accept your imperfect self, you will not abandon the child as he graphically shows you what you least like about yourself.

Anna sits in her office impatiently tapping the edge of the keyboard on her desk. Another hour and she can go home. She stares gloomily out the window at the office building across the street. How many women like her sit at their desks right now, waiting for the workday to be over? What are they thinking about in the meantime? The documents in front of them? Or their children? She imagines that there are mothers behind every window of the office building, mothers who are as skilled and confident at looking after their children as they are at their paid jobs. The standard of mothers is high these days, she believes. They all seem so competent. They put a lot of effort into providing their children with the best. A gust of envy passes through Anna. What about herself? Does she belong among these women? She quickly brushes away her concern. If all these women have succeeded, so will she. After all, she has worked her way up by her own accomplishments to the eight floor with her very own view of hundreds of other executives. What does she have to worry about?

Anna drops her hands down onto her lap and smiles to herself. What does Miriam care about pressure and competition? So far she gets what she needs regardless of what goes on in her mother's mind. How easy the first days of existence must be. Conversely, Anna must admit, motherhood is also easy at this point. But this peaceful state is soon over. Then what?

Anna's patience is running thin. What does she really know about what lies ahead? When will she have grasped what it means to be a mother? Right now, she feels, right now is an important moment. She is going to learn the art of mothering, and it is going to happen right now.

Anna continues to stare emptily in front of her. She has a strange feeling that she is being watched. Someone seems to be staring at her from deep inside the computer screen on her desk. When Anna looks closely she can make out the contours of a dark face outlined against the orangetoned screen. It is the face of an old woman. Her skin has lines like the bark of a pine tree and the same tan color. The lean face has deep hollows that hold two piercing eyes. Anna watches how the old woman's dry lips stretch across her cheekbones before they contract to form words:

"Here you sit, Anna, daydreaming about motherhood as usual," her voice heckles. "What a waste of time! It is time to act now, my friend. How else are you going to be a good mother for your child?"

Anna does not answer. This is the first time someone has appeared inside her computer screen. She ought to scream. Who is this grotesque woman Anna has never met before but who seems to know her so well? What does she want? Why is she here?

"I am here to make sure you learn the secrets of motherhood. I am very wise and I can do magic. Listen carefully to what I have to say. I can be very helpful to you. I have seen more women than you can ever imagine end up the way you so highly desire. I can transform you into the Perfect Mother in no time!"

Anna lightens up. Suddenly the answer to her agonies seems to have appeared right before her eyes. A fast and easy way to become a good mother is just what she is after. This woman seems to understand Anna and her predicament. Surely this is a woman she can do business with!

"The price?" The old woman sounds somewhat vague. "My advice will of course cost you, but my price is fair. I prefer to look at this as a mutually rewarding transaction. You will give me what I need, and in return you will gain what you stubbornly sit here and yearn for."

Anna swallows the tiny "but" at the tip of her tongue, straightens herself up, and fixes her eyes as deeply into the screen as she can manage.

"Let's get started!" the crone wheezes enthusiastically. She shapes her hands into a bowl, which she extends toward Anna. "Now, first I want you to give me your tears, my friend. I am sure you can do without them."

"Why do you want my tears?" Anna asks, surprised.

"I have never had any. Besides, they are not good for your disposition, Anna. Tears can overflow and blur your vision as a mother. Now give them to me and all your irritating self-doubts will disappear. Without tears, you will not even be able to feel the loss."

Anna lets her tears fall. In the cup of the old woman's bony hands they turn into glittering silver.

"Ah!" the old woman exclaims. "Good girl. See how beautiful your vulnerability turned in my hands. So precious to me, so harmful to the Perfect Mother."

"Let's move on," the crone cries impatiently. "Let me have the warm blood of your womb that goes to monthly waste. Oh, do not worry about missing it; nowadays there are plenty of pills to take should you want more children. It is a brew that you can do without, I promise. Think of the nuisance it is. It makes you so temperamental and intense, even inspires you to talk nonsense about being connected to the moon and earth and believe you know without anything to show for it. Such hocus-pocus will only confuse you as a mother. You must be able to think clearly to comprehend motherhood."

Drop by drop the thick blood drips and the old woman catches it carefully. She shivers in excitement when the drops turn into glowing rubies in her hands.

"I don't understand," Anna says. "And when am I getting my part of the bargain?"

"Soon enough. Look, let me show you. The cloak I wear over my shoulders will soon be yours. Now, is that not exciting!"

Anna examines the cloak. It is made of thick gray sacking, sewn together with leather strips to a foot-long coat. How ugly it is. And how heavy it looks. The cloth is very dense. It will not let anything breathe through.

"It is a little bit uncomfortable at first. But bear with it. As long as you carry this cloak only the very best way to mother can pass through its shield."

"Nobody will recognize me in this," Anna says doubtfully.

"You will be envied by everyone. No other woman has a cloak as useful as this one. Everyone will admire how effortlessly it all comes to you. You will be the Perfect Mother. They will all desperately try to imitate your style. But listen now to my last request from you. It is a mere trifle. It will not be any sacrifice at all."

"Then what do you ask from me?" Anna wonders, happy that the deal will soon be completed.

"Actually, my request comes as a bit of advice. Will you please show you are an adult now, Anna? Grow up, and do it at once! You must immediately stop daydreaming, Anna. Give me your dreams, Anna! Give me your imagination! Give me your youthful soul!"

"Yes, this is what I am like," Anna whispers. "How can I be responsible for a child?"

Anna blows her soft breath onto the old woman. A child appears in the arms of the witch, an infant swaddled in a plaid of silver and red rubies. A golden aura surrounds the child as it lies peacefully asleep. It is the most beautiful child Anna has ever seen.

At the same moment Anna feels a slow rumbling in her belly that ripples across her womb like a wave washing over the seashore. The sensation is new and wonderful and yet so familiar. How she has been waiting for this moment! Anna is startled to her senses.

"No!" Anna screams and takes the golden baby away from the old woman's arms. "I won't do it!"

A furious roar lingers in the air as Anna watches the computer screen flash and then go blank. Anna sits with her eyes closed until the panic slowly loses its grip. When she finally looks at the computer again there is nothing there but her unfinished document.

Pay attention to the quickening. Feel how the first fluttering sensation grows and spreads until it ripples strong and clear over the surface of your belly and there is no longer any doubt that there is life inside you. The Golden Baby is present and she will not be sold to the Perfect Mother. She will help you transform your selfcritical voice to a voice full of laughter and life.

Let the quickening point to the graceful center deep down in your womb where you can relax and be at ease, knowing that you will grow into your mother-self in your own time and way. Deep inside you will find your sincerity. The movement in your womb is secured to your willingness to try the best you can for the new life within. This is where your commitment to motherhood lies.

Chapter 3

A WOMAN'S WAY OF MOTHERING

The activities of pregnancy, birth, and mothering call upon the parts of our beings that are distinctly womanish. As a *pregnant woman* you prepare to animate the world with new life. You incite, vitalize, and vivify. You use your female body to imbue new life. You are part of the creative process in which life evolves and renews itself. Giving birth invites the resonant participation of our feminine spirits.

The mothering experience is a bestial and visceral experience, bringing us close to our animal nature. Flesh meets fluid in birth and nursing. Mothering is also a sensuous activity, calling for sweetness and softness, touch and embraces, warmth and comfort. It is about being sensitive and attentive to subtleties and entails the kind of strength that comes from succumbing to the natural process of life—the yielding force that accomplishes by flowing with the process instead of fighting against or forcing the movement. Lastly, mothering is an experience that opens us up to give and to receive. We open our hearts to the newborn child and out pour our sweetest feelings. In the midst of such magnificent love, we feel our own divinity.

Spirited, loving, divine—these are lavish promises of what becoming a mother will do to us. We can look forward to living our new mothering lives to the fullest. Our daily lives will be filled with the new soulfulness that birthing a child inspires in us. This delightful expression of the feminine self is precisely what attracts many of us to the idea of mothering a child. In motherhood we hope to find a place to express the parts of our femininity that may not have found an outlet in other activities. Motherhood will be a chance to devote ourselves to nurturing relationships and give of ourselves without other ambitions than to love. Also, we hope to share with the uninitiated child what life hitherto has taught us about truth and illusion. In essence, motherhood is a golden chance to present to the world our own interpretation of what it means to be a woman.

It would seem that the gravitation in motherhood toward the feminine is a natural continuation of who we already are as women. Caring for a child would only refine our present use of our feminine qualities. Yet, for many women of today embracing our femininity is not such a trouble-free undertaking. The transformation to mother is accompanied by fear of the unknown. There is a sense of being lost, of not knowing quite who we are and what to do with ourselves.

Full expression of a woman's femininity belongs in her everyday life and not just during the short moment in time when she becomes a mother. Yet, many of us find little use for these qualities in our achievement-oriented existence. We build our strength on our rational and analytical skills. We strive to be productive and disciplined, since these are qualities our society associates with success. Unfortunately, the goals we strive for are achieved at the expense of the expression of our feminine selves. We harden our hearts and petrify our sensitivity; in essence we decry our propensities for mothering a child.

The chapters "Project Baby" and "The Perfect Mother" both illuminate the troublesome ways in which a woman's unease with the workings of her femininity is revealed in pregnancy. The woman who is preoccupied with making her pregnancy a successful project is functioning in a mode far removed from the elegance of her feminine nature. Her agenda is exclusively geared toward proving herself a triumphant mother. Perfectionism is likewise detrimental to a true connection to a woman's female self. When critical thoughts and obsessive behaviors threaten to overshadow a woman's transformation to mother, there is little left for the play and pleasure that should nourish her body and soul—and thus the child—in pregnancy. She is so intent on pursuing the image of the mother she wishes to be that she forgets to take in life as it is. Quietly the beauty of pregnancy passes her by.

As we soon shall see, motherhood may be pivotal in awakening us to our femininity. The event lets us clearly see the virtues of our womanliness as we can cultivate and learn about these endowments in relationship to our children. What was at first a generator of discomfort and anxiety turns out to be a treasure of wisdom and strength. In the end, we will better understand ourselves as women.

In this chapter, we will focus on the nature of the challenges that we face as women in the transformation to mother. We will paint a portrait of the Modern Woman and the particularities she brings into motherhood. We will discuss her relationship to her femininity and how this relationship can either facilitate her transformation to mother or make it more difficult.

FEMININITY FEARED AND FOUGHT

The janitor glances in through Anna's open door. Anna smiles at him.

"Sorry, I am in your way again," she says. "Just leave this mess for tonight. This is the last night you will see me sweating over this project, I promise."

It is nine thirty. The rose-tinted light coming in from the window lets her know that she has missed out on another beautiful summer evening. She should be sitting with Thomas on the incline in Durham Park, where you can watch the evening sun color the rooftops in pastel colors. On a clear evening like this you can see the ocean laid out like a thin glittering ribbon west of the city. But here she is, in the seasonless blandness of her air-conditioned office.

If she only could come up with another couple of viable alternatives for her proposal. She needs something catchy and unexpected that will satisfy her client. Something to add cream to a rather ordinary cake. The presentation is tomorrow. By 9:00 a.m., the pile of notes on her desk will lie clean-typed on the conference table along with her drawings. It will not be easy, but she knows she can do it. She quite likes pressure. Her best ideas come forth when she is chasing the deadline.

So far, pregnancy has not slowed her down. In fact, she has almost been more productive since she found out she was expecting. But it will not be long until she will be forced to slow down. She can feel the change coming. Miriam will kick in her uterus and before she knows it, she has spent a half hour thinking about her baby. But she is not ready to be carried away just yet. From now until birth, work is her priority.

Motherhood, historically the quintessence of womanhood, challenges us to examine the personal characteristics we have placed at the base of our female selves. There was a time when there was little difference in how a woman would define herself as a mother and as a woman. A woman's primary role was to be the caretaker in the family, and thus to be feminine meant to be motherly: a nurturing and caring woman. Nowadays women readily oppose such narrow definitions of womanhood. We use attributes reflecting our skills in engineering, long-distance running, gardening, or whatever else we are committed to, to describe what we consider important to our identities. Motherhood may still be a woman's top priority and greatest source of pleasure, but is rarely the only occupation determining how she views herself. Motherliness is but one of her many fine qualities as a woman.

Along with changes in the sexual roles of recent years, the concept of femininity has changed from basically meaning a woman's sexual attributes and her domestic functions to a less restricting but far more ambiguous meaning. Femininity can now refer to everything from a woman's psychological stamina and independent nature, to her mystic side or her intellectual pursuits and spiritual interests. The construct is remolded in the individual psyche to fit the woman's view of herself.

As psychologist Joyce Block[1] points out, asking a woman how her feeling of femininity has changed after she became a mother is like giving a Rorschach ink blot test. Each woman will project her own ideas of what femininity means to her and then respond in these terms. In this context, we will assume that femininity is expressed in the intelligence, emotional reactions, and behaviors women exhibit as a result of their experiences as women. In using this definition, we attempt to take women's own experiences into account. The uniquely female experience of carrying a child in one's body is a clear expression of a woman's femininity. Although motherhood by no means is an imperative for a woman to be feminine, it is an important source of knowledge about her female nature.

The assertion that our female nature is influential in determining the transformation to mother is difficult to deny but raises a red flag in the minds of many women. They associate this idea with the view that anatomy is destiny and that certain characteristics such as dependency and passivity are intrinsic to the female nature. In psychological theory, Sigmund Freud's penis-envy theory represents the deterministic view of women's biological nature. Classic psychoanalytic theory asserts that a woman's longing for a child is an attempt to compensate for her unfortunate defect of having been born without a penis, a fact that forever renders her inferior to men. Any worldly ambitions she may have are but futile attempts at mimicking men, who possess the desirable organ. From Freud's viewpoint, motherhood seems to be the only normal, anatomically correct way for a woman to express her femininity.

Objecting to the biological determinism, some radical feminists assert that there are no real differences between men and women. The differences we see are a function of the patriarchal values of our male-dominated society that devalue women and are aimed at keeping women away from power. Femininity and masculinity are thus meaningless constructs. Along the same lines, mothering is said to be a socially conditioned behavior and not an expression of a biological predisposition.[2]

Other theorists propose that there are indeed sexual differences in how men and women relate to and manipulate the world.[3] Women's unique intelligence is, however, poorly understood in our society and has not yet been accepted as equal to men's. Jungian followers provide us with yet another point of view. They propose that women's femininity represents not only the biological and cultural influences on our identities, but a third, universal, and archetypal dimension, *the feminine*, which influences the lives of both men and women.

As long as we are childless we can personally avoid the problematic issue of what role our feminine nature plays in shaping who we are and what we do. We can minimize the question of sexual differences by pursuing interests and ambitions that challenge old-fashioned beliefs of what women can and cannot do. We can consider ourselves feminine even if we are not especially nurturing and caring, and we can reject whatever feminine qualities do not fit our ambitions. If there indeed are any differences, they do not necessarily show up in our daily lives.

The day a woman chooses motherhood, the confusion and ambivalence surrounding her femininity can no longer be ignored. By choosing to mother a child, we are also choosing to put our female characteristics at the forefront. Not surprisingly, the transformation to mother provokes a profound identity crisis in most of us. Indeed, the crisis has the same intensity many women of past generations experienced when they, after the children had left home, asked themselves, If I am not a mother, then who am I? Our generation is more likely to ask, If I am not a working woman, then who am I and who cares?

THE IDENTITY CRISIS OF MOTHERHOOD

It is ten thirty. The wastepaper basket is full but I have nothing to show for it. If only I did not feel so awful. Nausea and evening blues do not belong in the corporate world. I am a woman who has outgrown her business suit and does not know whether to stay or leave. Where do I belong now? I am a stranger on my own turf.

Professional world, you nurtured my ambitions. You encouraged me to develop my talents. You took me seriously. I wanted to perform for you and show you my gratitude. Now it is time to let go. No longer am I a true reflection of myself.

What lies next for me? I know I must search inside for the answers. But when I turn inside, I am no longer alone. I share myself with another. How will I then know who I am? Lest I am forever lost, I must know: How can I be a mother and myself?

Becoming a mother causes us to come to a full halt no matter how fast we are going. Stopped in our tracks, we are confronted with ourselves, as we really, truly are from the top of our heads to the souls of our feet. There is no polishing or refashioning allowed, no chance to hide behind well-rehearsed acting skills, no room for pretense or throwing blame around. This is it; this is what we have to work with. Here we have our own naked truth about ourselves, our givens and our potentials, ready to assert their influence on us as mothers and on our children.

Self-scrutiny is typical of pregnancy as we try to grasp the interpsychical and interpersonal ramifications of motherhood. The biological and psychological changes serve as an invitation to take a good look at ourselves and to ask where we stand on our chosen path in life. We come to ask ourselves difficult questions: *Who am I and where am I going? How will motherhood affect me? How will I change and in what ways will I remain the same? How can I be a mother and be myself?*

As Joyce Block points out, the transformation to mother is a careful balancing act between continuation and change in how we perceive ourselves.[4] Until we actually have experienced ourselves as mothers it is not clear exactly what will remain and what will change. We are in the midst of a spiritual birth, where life as we have known it is over, and the new life has not yet begun.

We do not part with what we define as essential to ourselves without stress and duress. Who is to say that we will not lose the parts of ourselves we hold dear, be it our freedom, youthfulness, or career interests? Worse yet, an unsettling feeling inside warns us that we may lose something even more fundamental and necessary to our well-being—that vague, ethereal, but oh so important sense of self. If pregnancy itself is an indication of the changes entailed, it is obvious that we are not talking pebbles and pennies here. You do not have to be far into pregnancy to realize that you are growing and changing faster than you can keep up with. How much can you reasonably change in nine months without losing grip on who you are?

The psychological changes of pregnancy and motherhood have been described as a crisis of intrapersonal and interpersonal disequilibrium and reorganization (Olds et al.),[5] a developmental stage (Duvall),[6] a shock (Harrison),[7] a series of transformative moments and themes (Bergum),[8] and a psychological genesis (Boroff Eagan).[9] These are dramatic descriptions of such a common event in women's lives as bearing a child. The transformation to mother is indeed a turning point in a woman's life bearing all the signs of a significant identity crisis.

The mother-to-be will reevaluate herself in relation to her past, present, and future. She will experience changes in such important contributors to her self-image as her marital relationship, occupational role, and social activities. She will reasses her past from her new perspective as a parent and incorporate her findings into her present self-image, and she must include the parent role in her plans for the future.

A woman's abilities to cope with these stressful changes is affected by such factors as whether the pregnancy was planned and desired, her general health and the health of the fetus in pregnancy, and the strength of the relationship with her partner. Socioeconomic status and availability of medical care and an adequate support system are other variables. Yet, even under ideal conditions, every new mother must expect to react with stress as she makes the necessary adjustments in her life.

The terminology used to describe the psychological changes of new motherhood previously reassures us that our struggles to come to terms with ourselves as mothers are indeed difficult but nevertheless common to pregnancy. We can give out a collective sigh of relief: Our unease is not a disease. Feelings of ambivalence, confusion, and distress are as intrinsic as physical complaints to the condition of pregnancy. The best we can do is to learn to cope with the inner turmoil the same way we learn to live with nausea and heartburn.

The identity crisis inherent in the process of becoming a mother is an especially pressing and difficult matter for women today. There is an urgency in our feelings of loss and confusion not experienced by previous generations. Whatever motherliness stands for in our minds it is something we do not easily embrace in ourselves. But why are our life-giving abilities so frightening to our female identities if we are dealing with normal psychological reactions to motherhood that any woman, regardless of what decade she lives in, will experience? In order to understand this peculiar situation, let us examine the characteristics of the Modern Woman, nineties style.

THE WAY OF THE MODERN WOMAN

In the corner of the window, right where Anna has put the folder that contains her project drawings, there sits a big, hairy spider. Anna stares at the creature, her damp hands clasping a firm ball of tissue paper. The spider stares back at her. Her eight arched legs are spread out around her fat belly, like a fleet of guards prepared to hurry her off swiftly in any direction. Anna stirs in her chair. The spider is motionless.

How ridiculous to be afraid of a spider, Anna tells herself. Just swat her with the paper and she will be gone. But Anna cannot bring herself to do it. An image of a black, hairy body, covered in blood and smeared into her palm, appears on her retina every time she gets ready to strike.

Anna glances at her watch. It is almost midnight. She cannot sit here and waste time anymore. She will just have to grab that folder and hope that the spider falls off. Darn spider. Why did she have to intrude upon her safe little world right now? This is an office on the eighth floor of a downtown architectural firm, not an abandoned log cabin in a forest.

The modern woman, as portrayed in media and literature, is a lady with backbone. She carries herself with a seemly posture that reflects inner determination and confidence—she has come a long way, baby, and she knows it. She has swiftly surpassed her female predecessors in educational and professional achievements and assured herself a position of influence in society. She has clear visions for what she wants to accomplish and confidence about achieving her dreams. She knows she is not the deficient Second Sex whose role is limited to sustaining the great advancers of civilization. She can strive, create, endure, and conquer as well as any man, and if women are not yet proportionally represented in positions of authority and power, it is not because they are inadequate to fill them but because the corporate glass ceiling stops their upward climb. In short, the modern woman defines herself in terms of her accomplishments and endeavors and values her independence and strivings for self-actualization.

As women have expanded their aspirations beyond the traditional roles of wife and mother they have developed sides of their personalities that previously were not associated with women. Women nowadays are as likely to characterize themselves as ambitious, dominant, and assertive as caring, soft, and compromising. The traditional ideals associated with women are often incompatible with what is rewarded in the world outside home. If a woman wants to assert herself in society, she is better off displaying herself as a female warrior rather than a softspoken princess.

Jungian-influenced writers and psychotherapists speak of women's current inclination to identify with the masculine principle of our society.[10] Our Western culture is structured around the masculine principle and favors objectivity, competitiveness, and productivity. A woman who seeks social recognition aside from the traditional role as caretaker must adapt these values and moderate her feminine qualities, including the parts of herself that are nurturing and feeling-based. Should she allow her feminine element to dominate she might be regarded as unfit to contribute to society in other ways than as wife and mother. Alternatively, she may choose to adopt the stereotypical image of femininity, aborting her need to develop her intellect and ambitions and adjusting her behavior to what pleases men.

In Jungian terminology, the masculine and the feminine are structures of our consciousness manifested in the emotional and behavioral responses of the individual and in images and symbols of our culture. The masculine principle analyzes, discriminates, separates, and controls. It is oriented toward ambition and goal achievement. An individual governed by the masculine principle favors a style of relating to others that emphasizes his need for separation and independence. On a collective level, the masculine element stands for law and order, technology, science, and cultural advancement.

The feminine principle, in contrast, unites, connects, absorbs, gestates, and yields.[11] The feminine is processoriented, that is, not concerned with the goal itself but with the process that leads to the goal. The striving toward wholeness is a major characteristic of the feminine as witnessed in "the desire to gather together, to patch things up, to unify seemingly disparate factors."[12] The feminine principle harbors an individual's capacity to connect and unite in relation to others, to bridge individual differences, and nurture their likeness.

The intelligence of the feminine element is intuitive, that is, capable of immediately understanding something without conscious reasoning. The feminine intelligence is also feeling-based and emotions are taken into account in decisions. Furthermore, the emotional and sensory acuity that comes from the body is an important foundation of the feminine. Collectively, the feminine concerns matter and earthiness as opposed to culture and is closely connected to the fecundity, fertility, and fruition of Mother Nature.

The feminine and masculine principles apply to both men and women, although we experience and relate to the two elements in different ways. A person, male or female, must have access to both the masculine and the feminine elements of the psyche in order to lead a rich soul life. The virtue of our inquiring and contemplative minds must, for example, be accompanied by full emotional recognition and expression. If either aspect is neglected, we become rigid and curbed in our actions and feelings. We then project our denigrated qualities onto others and become dependent on them to live out the attributes we do not recognize in ourselves.

Every woman brings her present self into her experiences of pregnancy and motherhood. A woman who is more comfortable with her masculine side will rely on her intellect to get the job done. For her, the most important task in pregnancy is to develop an understanding of the changes she is experiencing that is as comprehensive and helpful to her as possible. She is keen on acquiring as many facts as possible about what she can expect from pregnancy and motherhood. She strives for an objective outlook on the mother role, clarifying to herself what her own expectations are and what she can realistically expect from the experience.

The woman who operates out of the masculine principle views mothering as a set of behaviors she must learn. As for her pregnancy, she tackles aches and pains with logic and reason. If she attends birthing seminars or yoga classes she does so because she wants to broaden her understanding of pregnancy. She finds the right diet, physician, or birthing method to fit her particular beliefs. She is efficient, goal-oriented, and in control of her pregnancy.

In contrast, the woman who uses a feminine mode exclusively is content with directing her interest wherever her experiences in pregnancy will take her. It is more important for her to nurture her budding relationship with her child than to prepare for the future. Emotions guide her and can serve her well, as when she lets her feelings decide which caretaker she can build a trusting relationship with, or they can mislead her, as when fear keeps her away from preparing mentally for birth. She will attend birthing classes as a way to get the most out of her experience of pregnancy. She honors the ways of Mother Earth and makes her choices in accordance with her beliefs in nature's way.

In reality women are not as one-sided as in the two extreme examples given. Both the feminine and the masculine elements are present. The masculine approach is valuable in coping rationally with the anxieties of pregnancy and new motherhood. Our masculine side helps us to feel in control of our situation and not helplessly dependent on others to take care of us. The feminine element, on the other hand, gives us an instinctive understanding of mothering and an intimate connection to the child in the womb. Our feminine feeling for human relatedness lends profound meaning to our experiences and helps us endure even the toughest moments of pregnancy and motherhood.

THE LOSS OF FEMININITY

If a woman is so much more a woman when she is pregnant, how come I feel so lost? If I am doing what comes naturally to me, why am I so frightened?

I am in my most productive years: educated, experienced, and creative. Yet I did not create the child in my body. Life borrowed my womb. I am a woman, a vessel, passively waiting for life to unfold inside me.

Although the feminine side of a woman, particularly as described from a Jungian perspective, appears to be of great value to her, in reality few of us have learned to treasure its faculties. The feminine is part of the murky territories of our souls that we would rather not bother to associate ourselves with. Unwanted and unused, our womanliness appears increasingly more fearful to us. We declare the feminine aspect of our souls off-limits: the distrusted dark shadow of our self.

The loss of femininity is detrimental to the Modern Woman. A woman without her female spirit is a hollow character framed by pallor and aridity. Cut off from the needs and desires of her female self, she can only act from her whimsical ego. Her ambitions will reflect the values of society or influential persons in her surroundings rather than her own.

Since her accomplishments rarely are in tune with her inner self, they will not give her lasting satisfaction. She may appear strong and confident, but underneath the surface she feels inadequate. The woman may also lose touch with her emotional life. Rather than flowing with the richness of her shifting emotions, she is caught in an emotional state that is chronically deflated.

Family therapist Maureen Murdoch agrees that many women today are separated from their feminine nature. She says:

> In her desire to dispel the negative association with the feminine, our heroine has created an imbalance within herself which has left her scarred and broken. She has learned how to get things done logically and efficiently but has sacrificed her health, dreams, and intuition. What she may have lost is a deep relationship to her own feminine nature. She may describe and mourn the numbing of her bodily wisdom, the lack of time for family or creative projects, the loss of deep relationships with other women, or the absence if her own "little girl."[13]

As a result of suppressing their femininity, many women feel out of touch with themselves, harboring a gnawing sense of loss and betrayal in their hearts that interferes with their spiritual well-being. Unless they fill their inner emptiness with activity, they fall into melancholy. In order to regain a positive connection to the feminine, Murdoch says, women must embark on an inner psychological quest, *The Heroine's Journey*. Murdoch describes the spiritual journey as a spiral movement in which a woman becomes conscious of the value of her feminine nature and eventually heals her inner wounds.

The loss of the feminine is a problem among men and women alike. It is reflected not only in the individual but in our Western way of life. Jungian analyst Robert A. Johnson[14] argues that our culture is strongly one-sided in favor of the masculine principle. Our society is rich in technological and material progress but spiritually and emotionally impoverished. We are lacking in such noble values as warmth, contentment, and serenity. The feminine belongs to the shadow side of our culture, the unaccepted side which we keep at bay with severe social sanctions for those who dare to express its teachings. We see irrationality and malice in the feminine instead of beauty and enchantment.

Anna decides to leave the spider where it is. She cannot bring herself to kill it. She finally grabs the folder and the spider darts off and into a crack in the window frame. Anna returns to her work, keeping an eye on the spider every now and then. She half expects the spider to leap down on her desk and come toward her on her quick legs. But the spider sits quietly in her hideout.

Anna has back pains. She cannot continue like this. She must lie down for a while. She kicks off her shoes and lowers herself to the floor, slowly rolling over on her back.

Like a beetle, she thinks. A beetle stranded on its back, legs helplessly reaching into the air. An easy catch for a spider. Anna is not surprised to see that the spider has come out of her den. But she does not seem to be interested in Anna. She is moving back and forth in a complex pattern, spinning a delicate web with her sticky silk thread.

Suddenly Anna realizes how tired she is. She yawns and stretches her stiff body. She will just close her eyes for a few minutes. She can feel Miriam stirring inside her body. Is she perhaps amused by her mother's frenzy?

The tragedy of the loss of feminine values is never as paramount as in the way we approach motherhood. The very same attributes we have come to despise and associate with female inferiority are needed in mothering: Mothers nourish; mothers soothe; mothers yield to the needs of their children; mothers act on their feelings. Mothers are *feminine*, and they get their strength from a place deep inside their feminine selves.

The Modern Woman sees this and she fears. She tries everything to minimize this fact: She is going to parent, not mother. Times have changed, she insists. Motherhood is different now. She is not willing to compromise her identity for motherhood. Yet, despite her efforts to cover up the truth, the conflict surrounding her femininity is laid open.

Becoming a mother can be identified with few of the characteristics the Modern Woman values. Motherhood involves an infringement on her freedom and independence, a certain sacrifice of her ego drives and ambitions. It limits her capacities for social and occupational commitments and puts her in the unglamorous situation of having to focus on the basics at home. No matter how large a chunk of the responsibilities her spouse may assume, she cannot get around the fact that the activities of nurturing and caring will take up a major chunk of her daily life, in emotional involvement as well as in time.

For the independent, ambitious woman of our times such a radical change in priorities may seem a costly sacrifice. There are no guarantees that the mother role will not put her in the exact situation she has always feared: being chained to the destitution of her female nature. Will she now have to say good-bye to her freedom and power as a woman? Is this the end of the delightful era of self-respect she has found in her masculine demeanor?

The fear that the mother role will negatively affect a woman's sense of self appears to be confirmed by pregnancy. Measured against the yard stick of her female ideals, the psychological changes the pregnant woman experiences seem to work against her. Emotionally labile, absentminded, and having concentrating difficulty, the pregnant woman has seemingly lost her intellectual edge. Especially during the latter part of pregnancy, many women are less able to cope with stress and become irritable and tense in the face of even minor frustrations. The pregnant woman also frequently feels extra need for attention and care from others, a blow to her valued autonomy.

Later on, the realities of motherhood may also make a woman doubt the survival of her former competent self. Weak and fatigued, she has trouble dealing with the simplest household tasks. Being tied to home gives rise to feelings of isolation and loneliness. The step is small for her to believe that the personal transformation has indeed been for the worse.

After birth, most women gradually overcome the dramatic feelings of the transition to motherhood and return to a more favorable opinion of themselves. In fact, many new mothers report that motherhood has brought them closer to their ideal selves.[15] The competence that comes from coping with the new responsibilities and the feeling of being so utterly important to your child enhance the self-esteem.

In order to reach these mothering heights, the Modern Woman must be prepared to work consciously toward a new appreciation of her femininity and explore how she best can connect with her inner self.

MOTHERHOOD AS A WAY TO EXPLORE OUR FEMININITY

My child, you are the life born out of my womanhood.
Kicking and turning in your borrowed space,
the space we share,
in which you are protected and at peace
while I am disquieted.
I have severed the lifeline
that yet keeps you unaware of yourself.
Knowledge sometimes makes for cowardice,
I have lost my innocence.
I look into the darkness of my womb,
expecting a reflection.
It is so dark
I can barely make out the contours of a woman
rising out of the waters.
She moves to the rhythm of pulsating blood,
a woman who has never listened to the dictates of culture.

To her, the womb is a world with no restrictions,
a sacred place, where you are free
to become what you were meant to be.
She calls me: Come and befriend the darkness!
She, who dares to search for what she has lost,
will find the wisdom of the womb.

In the prologue to *To Be a Woman—the Birth of the Conscious Feminine,* Connie Zweig argues that today, as "women are defined less and less by biology, and are growing less constrained by the idealized projections of men. . . . for the first time, the Feminine can become *conscious* in women—not male-identified, not in reaction to something other, not compensating for something missing."[16] Women thus have an opportunity to redefine and transform the feminine principle and to live a kind of femininity that, consciously chosen, breathes new life into our society. The new consciousness of the feminine is, in Connie Zweig's words, "like a root shooting up through the cracked concrete surface of the culture."

Many women have come to realize that their psychological strength is different from what society typically honors and that it does no good to try to conform to a male model of power and success. CEO, division manager, or major—a woman's goals will give her little satisfaction without the affirmation of her female self. As women increasingly have found ways to be strong and independent in the outer world, they see the need to free their psychological realities as well. Each woman must find her unique way of letting her female soul out.

Marion Woodman is among the women who have redefined the influences of our biological nature in positive terms. To Woodman, we will find the key to a positive relationship to our feminine selves in our bodies. The body mirrors a woman's soul. To be negligent of one's biological nature is "to be a soul in search of a body." Woodman says: "For the woman, at least, her identity is indistinguishable from her body, and until she learns to look at it as the nourishing source of her feminine identity she will remain out of touch with herself, wandering about in a world alien to her feminine ego."[17] If it is true that our bodies can put us back in touch with our feminine spirit, the bodily experience of pregnancy and birth promises to be a time of self-discovery and growth.

The riches a woman receives when she comes to experience her authentic femininity are abundant. Her female creativity can flow freely and add to her professional and private spheres alike. She may find new talents to pursue or refresh her ideas of present endeavors. She reconnects with her intuition and can use this power to protect and assert herself in the world. Her new spontaneity and ability to live in the moment revitalize her soul and change her attitude toward the inevitable mishaps of life. Relationships begin to bloom under her attention. She can work on achieving caring relationships with men and women that value both the differences and the similarities of the sexes. Grounded in her feminine nature, she can feel a new sense of inner peace and well-being.

We can easily understand how a woman who is consciously working on finding her feminine self may become interested in bearing a child. The process of such inner work bears many similarities to what happens in pregnancy. In her quest for psychological growth, the woman gives symbolic birth to herself. She comes to understand what it is like to be impregnated with an idea of spiritual magnitude and to recognize that pursuing this idea leads to profound inner transformation. She knows how patiently to carry her poetic child within until the child is ready to be born. She typically learns to put emphasis on fostering and nurturing whatever needs her devotion, whether it be her relationships, ideas and opinions, or physical body.

In this frame of mind, the woman readily connects with the young. Like children, she finds satisfaction in being, not only in doing. Children live close to their feelings, and so does she. She will pay special attention to her imagination and dreams, the same inclination that appears so naturally in children. Finally, she typically learns to pay attention to her female body and its importance to her well-being. The cyclicity of her reproductive system, the monthly repetition of fertility and barrenness, reminds her of her physical propensity for childbearing.

As a mother, a woman can continue to experiment with her femininity. Ultimately, the feminine and the masculine elements will be integrated. The mother learns how to use her creativity and assertiveness when she is nurturing her child, and to nurture her creativity and need for self-expression when she is out in the world.

There are many ways to express our feminine nature and childbearing is only one of them. Women who have been awakened to the subject typically gravitate toward many different ways of displaying their feminine selves. Women show who they are when they create poems and jewelry, when they dance and sing, when they voice their feminine ideals in politics, when they care for the environment-there are as many ways as there are individuals.

The growing interest in the female self is witnessed in the popularity of works that offer an expanded vision of what it means to be a woman. Books such as *Goddesses in Everywoman*[18] and *Women Who Run With the Wolves*[19] are instrumental in helping women find new aspects of themselves. There is also a nationwide interest in female spirituality. Women come together to develop their own understanding of spiritual matters and to find a form of worship that satisfies their feminine spirit. Research into ancient goddess cultures has inspired women to look at mother images more powerful than real-life mothers as sources of inspiration.[20] Likewise, psychotherapy and selfhelp groups provide forums for women to explore their female selves and to see their individual feelings and symptoms in a new context.[21]

Having a child remains for many the ultimate manifestation of their feminine powers. A woman can, consciously or unconsciously, make the choice to have a child either in an effort to regain the missing pieces of her feminine self or, better yet, in a celebration of her womanhood and willingness to share the experience of having a child with her mate. Either way, in accepting the mother role the woman implies she is no longer willing to let the negative qualities associated with that role prevent her from becoming a mother.

Chapter 4

WALKING IN MOTHER'S FOOTSTEPS

The flight attendant demonstrates the correct use of the oxygen mask. Anna, who rarely pays attention to the safety instructions, finds herself watching the stewardess's demonstration closely. What if the improbable occurs? What are the odds that the baby and she will survive a crash landing? Even if technology stands by them and they arrive safely, she is not sure it is wise to make this trip at seven months pregnant. Will the baby get enough oxygen at this altitude? What would happen if she suddenly went into premature labor? Or what if she is exposed to some strange virus and falls seriously ill? She should not have agreed to this trip. She should have stayed home. Nevertheless, here she is: A three hour plane ride and she will be back in her childhood surroundings, or rather, she will be surrounded by her past.

This time is different. She is pregnant. Her protruding stomach will prevent her from turning into young Anna again. She knows how it usually works: The first few days at home are fine. She enjoys her mother's pampering and her father's attempts at concealing his excitement at her arrival. The slow pace of rural Michigan relaxes her urban nerves and she wonders why she ever left. She sleeps late in the morning, eats her favorite foods, and takes relaxing walks. The shift creeps up on her slowly, but the day inevitably comes when she finds herself uncertain about her age; is she thirteen years old, or three?

Darn seat. Anna is so uncomfortable. Her legs hurt. The weight of the baby presses on her lower back. If only they will turn off the seat-belt sign so she can get up and stretch. And why do they never show up with the advertised refreshments? Anna turns in her seat. She should not have left. She should have insisted that her parents visit her instead. But her Dad does not like to travel since his heart attack and Elna refuses to leave him home alone. At least that is what she claims.

Anna goes over the phone conversation she had with her mother a couple of weeks ago when it became clear that her parents were planning a trip to the Caribbean for the two weeks following Anna's due date. They were sorry they would not be able to see the newborn baby, her mother had said, but this vacation was too good a deal to pass up. Anna unexpectedly burst into tears. How could they prefer going on a vacation to meeting their new grandchild? Anna could not hide her disappointment, no matter how embarrassed she felt at her childish outburst. Elna apologized and said that she had not realized they would leave right at the due date when she booked the trip, but now that she finally had convinced Ivar to go, they wished to stick to their plans.

Perhaps this was the truth, but Anna was not consoled. She could not help but think that her mother's decision (there was no doubt in her mind that the decision was her mother's) in fact reflected her feelings toward Anna. Elna was simply not all that interested in her becoming a mother. Anna's fertility threatened her; it was the final evidence that Anna no longer was her little girl, that she was a woman who in many ways had surpassed her mother and who now would encroach on her mother's domain.

Pregnancy awakens many thoughts and feelings about your own mother, a person who no doubt will have great impact on your transformation to mother. Suddenly you feel subtle pulls in the umbilical cord that, although invisible, tie the two of you together. Whether well-filled and nourishing or dried-out and brittle, this emotional cord determines that the two of you belong together. The umbilical cord assures that part of your relationship will always be defined as that between a mother—the older and more experienced woman—and her daughter—the younger recipient of her mother's wisdom and love.

The umbilical cord is never severed once and for all. It continues to live within the psyche of every woman and will influence and guide her thoughts and actions, often unconsciously, as she enters into motherhood. Attending to the mother-daughter relationship is an important aspect of the inner work of becoming a mother. The psychological task is to find comfort in the emotional ties to one's mother, while establishing oneself as a new mother. Although inexperienced, each of us is entitled to mother differently than our mother.

A WOMAN'S FIRST MOTHERING EXPERIENCE

Your mother gave you your first and most important lesson in motherhood. Although your father and others also influenced you to become who you are, in motherhood it is nevertheless your mother whom you will most resemble. She is the one in whose footsteps you are walking. You once watched very closely as she performed and imitated her in your play so that you one day could be like her. These childhood observations now form the foundation for your own parenting style, how you perceive yourself as a parent, and how you relate to your child. Moreover, as a child you were not only an observer of your mother's life but the impetus for her parenting efforts. You were utterly dependent on her as the source of love and closeness, guidance and encouragement, and, as the years went by, as the person to defy and criticize and eventually leave.

Out of your childhood relationship with your mother grew your sense of self. Jungian analyst James Hillman puts forth:

The way we feel about our bodily life, our physical self-regard and confidence, the subjective tone with which we take in or go out into the world, the basic fears and guilts, how we enter into love and behave in closeness and nearness, our psychological temperature of coldness and warmth, how we feel when we are ill, our manners, taste, and style of eating and living, habitual structures of relating, patterns of gesture and tone of voice, all bear the marks of mother.[1]

We build our sense of self, our ability to love ourselves and believe in our own worth independent of what others think, out of our mother's love and care. Our estimation of what we can do with ourselves, how far we can reach, and how high we should aim also comes from watching our mothers carry out their lives.

Your personal assessment of your experiences with mother greatly affects how you will relate to your expanding feminine self as you become a mother. Your mother was the first feminine figure in your life and what she taught you about being a woman affects your emotional and spiritual growth to this day. Your experience in her care determines whether you will welcome your new feminine side as it reveals itself in the mother role or whether you will feel chilled to the bones. If your mother was able to love and nurture her children passionately and enjoyed doing so, you will expect motherhood to be fun and rewarding; if she harmoniously divided the care with your father, you will see shared parenting as the way to go; and if she had rewarding interests outside of the mother role, you will find it natural to take on other projects. In essence, you will have learned not to fear your nurturing side, because your mother showed you how mothering can enhance a woman's sense of self rather than cause her to lose her identity. Conversely, if your mother failed to provide you with the basics of love and recognition, you will be uncertain in your own abilities to give sufficiently to your child; if she was depressed and bitter, you will have to work hard to prove that maternity can be a rewarding experience; and if she did not realize other ambitions aside from taking care of you, you may fear that the mother role will put an end to your abilities to enjoy the outside world.

Every daughter must eventually leave her mother's protective embrace to find her separate identity. En route to independence we are often more interested in the ways we are different from our mothers than in our similarities. It may at times seem that there is little we have in common with the woman who bore us. In fact, we may pride ourselves on our dissimilarity and use the differences we discover to enhance our feelings about ourselves: "At least I am not as low paid, bored, manipulative, or ignorant as my mother!" the adult daughter exclaims in relief. In the individuation process, the cord between mothers and daughters often becomes clogged with sediments of faultfinding and blame that will restrain rather than further our development as mothers. It seems as if we are collectively stuck in this youthful stage of criticism. We habitually blame and pity our mothers for the way they carried out the mother role. "Mother" stands for a victimized woman, who lives a life in stagnation. Our negative associations not only make it difficult for us to accept our likeness to our mothers but also prevent us from taking advantage of the customs and knowledge the older generation possesses.

TO BECOME A MOTHER IS TO BECOME LIKE YOUR
MOTHER

Pregnancy marks the beginning of a significant change in your relationship to your mother. From now on you and your mother will be able to relate to each other on more equal terms as two women who share the experience of motherhood. You have an opportunity to discover each other once more and to tie a new bond between you, beyond the original cord. Motherhood may be the first time that you can truly identify with your mother's life as a parent. Here is a woman who once was just as unsure and inexperienced as you are. She learned about the love, pain, and worries of mother-hood, the universal truths about having children, just as you will. You may be struck by how much responsibility your young mother had, how hard she had to work, and how little time she had to herself. Her crazy ways of treating you that you have criticized so fiercely suddenly seem reasonable or at least understandable. From this new understanding of her role, you will theoretically be able to look at your mother with renewed fondness and respect.

Pregnancy can inspire you to a closer and more democratic relationship with your mother, which in turns shifts how you relate to yourself, but the transition will also blow new life into any negative feelings you harbor. Whatever frictions there have been will resurface, whether they be harmless disputes over all those minor injustices she once inflected upon you or painful recollections of abuse and neglect. Conse-quently, you may either resent mother's involvement in your pregnancy and fear that her presence will influence you in negative ways or, like Anna, wonder about her lack of involvement and wish that she would participate more.

It is a questionable pleasure to discover the ugly little vermin inside that gnaw away at our wish to be undividedly happy as new mothers. In many ways it would be much easier if we mentally and emotionally were freed of our past when we gave birth. With a clean record and a short memory we could immerse ourselves in the mother role with immediate success. However, pregnancy is a sure sign that we have lost our innocence. We are old enough to know that, for better or worse, our personal histories remain with us and will be faithfully revived when we become parents.

The remedy to simply repeating our past with our children, and with ourselves, lies in our willingness to look back and examine how our early relationships have influenced us to become who we are and continue to influence us in the present. Without these insights we are likely to stumble into similar situations with our children that will undermine our happiness as mothers. Comprehension is our chance to see problems between us and our children as they develop and take action before events get out of hand.

FACING YOUR AMBIVALENCE

"Taking a closer look at my relationship with Mother is sensible," Anna thinks. "It's important. It will help me become a better parent. Then again, I really have better things to do with my time. Besides, it is such a worn-out subject. What else was

I brooding upon as a teenager, and well into my adult years as well? I know my old childhood traumas forward and backward, and they do not excite me anymore. Why dig up old material again? I should be happy and harmonic when I am pregnant, and not sit and ponder profundities. I am sure it will affect the child."

Sometimes it is difficult for a woman to acknowledge her mother's influence in motherhood. Many adult daughters interpret independence and self-reliance to mean that they should refuse any support. They would rather risk standing without help than admitting that they are not fully autonomous. "Why should I not figure out motherhood on my own?" a woman may reason. "I am an adult now and can take care of myself. Mother was important when I was young and helpless, but why should I need her now?" Mother's merits may also be questioned: "What does she know about disposable bottles, infant exercise regimens and the best child care in town? Her expertise is history and hardly suitable for my contemporary baby. I must break away from tradition and find my own way."

Although it is true that the mother role has changed significantly, there are many aspects of motherhood that remain the same. Giving birth signals a profound change in women's lives, independent of what time and age they live in. Babies must be held, fed, and loved no matter what. Your mother has the clear advantage in this situation of having experienced what it takes to care for someone as young as you once were.

The mixed feelings most of us have toward our mothers make it difficult to look at this relationship without hesitation. No one was born with the ideal mother as her biological mother. As it is in the ordinary mother's nature to misunderstand and make mistakes, we have all from time to time been hurt as children. The extent and severity of these afflictions vary greatly and will naturally determine how easy it will be to focus on the present relationship. In this there is no fairness. As tempting as it may be to ignore the mayhem that arises when we delve into the past, understanding what has formed our expectations is a necessary part of resolving any difficulties we have in adjusting. Many of our unrealistic expectations about motherhood make sense when we examine them from the perspective of our earliest attachments, as do our doubts and ambivalence.

Your mother can be part of your preparations for motherhood whether the two of you have personal contact or not. Her participation can take place entirely in your mind. You can reflect on your relationship in private and remind yourself what it was like to be her daughter and how you envision mothering from her perspective. Asking yourself about the strengths and weaknesses of her ways, what you would like to adopt yourself and what you want to do differently, helps you to clarify your own ideas about motherhood. From your new perspective as a mother, you will reassess your mother's impact on your life and most likely experience a change in the way you think of her.

Insight into days gone by is not sum total of what we should look for in our mothers. We also need our mothers in a way that is less threatening than examining their impact on our lives can be. We need to look to our mothers for inspiration and strength. We need to look to our mothers as women who can tutor us in an art that we have yet to master: the art of using our womanly capacities to mother, and to mother in a healthful way that will enliven both ourselves and our children.

In becoming mothers, we have a choice to continue to believe that our mothers either were completely unimportant or totally detrimental to who we now are or we can approach her with a whole new set of ideas and questions: We can use our mothers to understand ourselves better as women and to uncover the pieces so many of us have set aside or lost in our pursuit of fame and fortune. Although our mothers most likely will not be able to give us the full scope on how a woman is to make good use of her nurturing side, we can at least find clues in their vicinity.

Recognizing the good that comes from examining the relationship with our mothers, let us now take the frightened and protesting child within by her hand and carefully approach what once was.

THE ORIGINAL CORD: MOTHER THROUGH THE EYES OF THE CHILD

Anna opens the door to her old room upstairs. Her mother has not remodeled in here. Nothing has changed since Anna left. The room is like a museum, a historical monument of Anna Theresa Biorck's childhood years, preserved for posterity by Elna Biorck, her mother. Anna alternatively ridicules and takes delight in her mother's refusal to make alterations and accept that her daughter now is out of her hands.

Anna quietly closes the door behind her. She wants to be alone on her journey back in time. Awkwardly she lowers herself to the floor. From this perspective it is easier to see what young Anna once saw. Tiny pink roses bloom eternally on the walls, and the green carpet stretches like a spring lawn in front of her. The many posters covering the blooming walls reveal that Anna eventually outgrew the girlish cuteness of the room's interior. She had done her best to cover the flower patches with posters of galloping horses, rock stars, and famous athletes. One side of the wall displays four brown glue stains in a square formation. The poster of four bare-chested men in black leather that adorned this place vanished quietly as soon as Anna moved out of the room.

The white four-poster bed was once Anna's pride. Anna smiles nostalgically as she remembers the squeaking protest the bed springs let out as you sunk into the depths of the mattress. In this bed many dreams had been woven. Here Anna had lain in the shelter of the dark night and fantasized about such topics as an upcoming school dance, her future as a famous TV reporter, an adventurous trip across the plains of Australia. Here her girlfriends gathered to make confessions about their latest love interests, the details and subsequent analyses changing drastically over the years. In the cushioned shelter of her bed the world had seemed wide open and their courage and deftness to conquer this world unlimited.

What is on top of the bed? Propped up against the head pillows is a doll, dressed like a Raggedy Ann in red and white stripes, one arm missing and the other oddly twisted behind her back. Where on earth did Elna find this doll? She had no idea her mother had bothered to keep her for this long. Why did she take the trouble to bring her out of the closet right now when Anna was pregnant? What did she want to convey to her daughter with this gesture?

Anna carefully picks up Rosita-Louise. Her chubby plastic legs dangle lifelessly from her body. Anna counts her toes. She notices that each toe has a tiny pink toenail and painted skin folds at the joints. Anna studies the doll's face. Her marzipan skin is soft and blemish-free. The pink lips protrude around the dark hole awaiting the baby bottle. Two bright eyes stare intently at Anna, watching her appealingly, yearningly. Before Anna knows it, the burning lump in her throat bursts and ridiculous, crude tears roll down her face. With Rosita-Louise against her chest she gives in to her shaking body.

Once upon a time there was a little girl whose name was yours. She had the best mother in the whole world, this she knew for sure. Her mother made the best noodles and from her milk cartons flowed the sweetest milk. She could count to fifty-eleven at least, and she always knew when it was time for you to play, eat, and sleep. She understood exactly what was the matter when you came running in with squirting tears or when you sat tight-lipped on the sofa. With a kiss and some magic words she made everything all right again. She loved you more than anything, even more than she loved Dad and your silly younger brother. She was always there to hold you, listen to you, and explain the mysteries of life to you. When you grew up you wanted to be just like her.

"Stop it!" you moan. "My childhood was not like that at all. I remember mother's bad side just as clearly. She was not the best mother in the world; I knew this perfectly well. Why not? Well, she dragged me to ballet classes although I hated classical music and dusty wood floors. When my brother bicycled across the living room she laughed hysterically, but when I repeated the act she threw a fit. She made me eat spinach even though it turned my stomach. She smiled falsely at my attempts at poetry, and demanded I help her with housework instead. While I was still young and helpless she abandoned me for a new job. And she failed to prepare me for life: she left me all confused and naive to handle the pitfalls of adulthood on my own."

Both of these mother images, the good mother and the bad mother, belong to the child. As children, we have our own way of looking at reality. We believe that everything that happens centers around us. The world is magical and our mother and father are the omnipotent rulers of this incomprehensible world. Whatever mother does, she does for our sake. We divide her actions into good and bad: they are intended either to please or to hurt us. We fail to see that mother's actions can be motivated by factors that have little to do with us.

The glorified "good mother," who is loving, wise, and always available, is deeply rooted in our souls, and this for some very good reasons. As children we need to believe in the benevolence of our caretakers since we are utterly dependent on their care. Our conviction of our parents' goodness and omnipotence gives us an important foundation for a positive self-image: If my mother is good and loving, and I am her beloved child, then I must be good and lovable. In psychological terms, we *internalize* the good mother, and hence gain confidence in ourselves. So important are our parents to us that we will adulate their behaviors even when they are clearly destructive to our well-being. The abused child will often defend his parent's actions rather than blame them and will believe that the abuse is his rightful punishment for being a bad child. In order to survive in a psychological sense, we cannot believe other than that our parents know best.

The image of the ideal mother from which we built our self-esteem as children is also important for our adult well-being. The internalized good mother is a source of security and support that we can retreat to when the pressures of the adult world are overwhelming. The mother within exists purely for our psychological prosperity. She is an eternal reservoir of feminine strength who is there to give us comfort and support when we need her.

Our real mothers rarely live up to the idealized image of the good mother, nor should we expect them to. As adults we can tolerate and sympathize with their imperfections, knowing that we no longer are dependent on them for our inner sustenance. We can find for ourselves what we need in order to grow and thrive as women. As adults we can also choose to model the image of the good mother after women other than our biological mothers. We may find a human counterpart of the good mother in the form of nurturing relationships with close friends, the extended family, or perhaps a therapeutic relationship. We may also find her to be of a purely etherieal presence, as when we are nurtured and inspired by a religious faith or by Mother Nature. It is our image of the good mother rather than our real mother who becomes our guiding light in motherhood.

THE ORIGINAL CORD AND THE FUNDAMENTALS OF MOTHERING

Our mothers, who in our generation most often were our primary caregivers, helped us develop the inner strength we now need to become good and loving parents. We can single out four different ways in which our mothers promoted our psycho-emotional development and thus laid the groundwork for our own abilities to mother. The first and foremost of these fundamentals of mothering are mother love and the nurturing and protective activities that spring forth from this love. The experience of being loved provides us with the raw material for a healthy sense of self. Nancy Friday writes:

> Healthy, primary narcissism is rooted in infancy. Mother is the first "objective" voice we hear; her face is our first mirror. When we are born, she cannot hear enough wonderful things being said about us. She absolutely absorbs the praise of friends and relatives as they coo and gurgle about our beauty, size, and amazing agility. She transfers it to us like heat. At this stage she is rightly so tied to us that she does not know where praise for us leaves off and admiration for her giving birth to such a miraculous baby begins. We feed her narcissism and she feeds ours. It is the height of symbiosis at its best, primary narcissism functioning as it should. Our ego is born.[2]

If we have received our parents' love, we will develop trust in ourselves and in our own worth that will help us through the difficulties of life with our sense of self intact.

We may temporarily lose our bearings, as may happen in the first confusing months of new motherhood, but in the end we will find our way back to a positive feeling about ourselves. Healthy narcissism, "that tidal basin out of which all maternal emotions flow," is essential to loving an infant. Out of our love and acceptance of ourselves come our feelings for the child.

The second of the fundamental principles of mothering is adequate mirroring: the process in which a mother reflects back to the daughter who she is. The child looks at her mother and finds affirmation for her feelings and reactions reflected in her mother's face. The more a mother can accept and affirm in her child without judgment or distortion (and this means her talents as well as her difficulties, her plainness as well as her extraordinariness) the more there will be of her child's sense of self. A self once enhanced in a straightforward way acquires capital stock in the transformation to mother. If we have learned that all of our feelings and behaviors are acceptable, we will have few problems embracing both our strengths and our limitations as young mothers. Emotionally, we can handle the ambivalent feelings of pregnancy and motherhood without getting stuck in self-blame and guilt. We carry a basic trust in our own goodness, no matter what we are feeling in the moment. And if we have learned to accept ourselves, we can in turn accept our own children as they are.

Third, we need our mothers to have been good role models for us, both in the mother role and as women in their own right. No matter how sincerely our mothers encouraged us to find our own way, and no matter how different our lives and values now are, we still will feel most comfortable when we follow in their footsteps. How they actually lived their lives matters more than any advice and hindsight they may offer by mouth. If, for example, mother successfully managed to balance career and homemaking, we will feel free to do the same. On the other hand, if the mother never worked outside the home, we may find it difficult to justify leaving our children in someone else's care.

The power that our early identifications have on our outlook on motherhood can also play havoc with us by compelling us to repeat our mother's misjudgments. Outwardly we seem to arrange for situations that are radically different from our mother's lives, but when it boils down to it we may discover that there are many similarities. If mother lived a restricted life and was depressed as a result, we may ourselves fail to take advantage of our chances to be happy, and even if no complications or other circumstances cloud pregnancy, we may still identify with mother's resentment and dislike being pregnant or fall into bouts of depression.

Lastly, our mothers are our seeresses, not because they possess the ability to see into our future, but because the legacy of their own lives suggests to us what we can expect from our future as mothers. Our eyewitness account of their joys and pains in motherhood is our most trustworthy record of what it will be like to have children. If mother enjoyed having children to look after, so will we most likely. We expect our children to be well worth the effort we must put into their care. If, on the contrary, we believe that mother resented her caretaking role, we may well be afraid to fall into the same unfortunate situation.

THE ORIGINAL CORD AND THE TRANSFORMATION TO MOTHER

"Mom, why did you bring out my old doll? Do you think I need to practice being a mother on her?"

"Good heavens, no. I don't think you need to practice. You will know what to do, as every mother does. I was just looking through some old boxes and there she was, the only doll that ever could compete with your interests in ballgames and bicycling and treeclimbing. You really did not care much for dolls, you know."

"That is exactly what worries me, how I never liked those pretend games of cuddling and feeding dolls, and I sometimes think that, perhaps, I will be as indifferent to my child as I once was to them."

"Don't be ridiculous. You don't feel indifferent to that little creature kicking inside you this very minute, do you? Of course you will love your child."

"You make it seem as if there is nothing to mothering a child. You give birth just like that, you look at your infant, and then you pick up where you left off the day you last played with your dolls as a child. You do not understand how I feel."

"You are still mad at me for that Caribbean trip, are you not?"

"No, I don't care; I think you should go, but, well, I mean yes, I think it is a rotten thing to do to me. For all these years you have practically begged me to allow you to care for me like I was a little girl again, but now when I actually need you, you decide to go on a vacation. What am I to make out of it? You act like a vengeful Demeter to me."

"For goodness sake, Anna, stop seeing me as a useless old hag! You can never forgive me for loving to be a mother the way I did, can you? Why, Anna? What is so terrible about being a mother? I would have hoped that now when you finally have chosen to have a child yourself you would come to view me in a different light. You are fighting me all the way, yet like me you will be. Honestly, it hurts me to see you reject all that I was to you. And I am worried about you. I wonder, how will this girl be able to find grace in motherhood? Well, Anna, you might find it hard to believe, but I see how you struggle, and when I put Rosita-Louise on the bed for you to find I secretly hoped that you would remember how you once loved and cared for her. You would not believe me if I told you outright that you will be a wonderful mother, but I hoped that by remembering the girl you once were, you would be reassured. Truthfully, that was my intention when I put the doll on your bed."

Colors mix inside Anna. Red and brown, yellow patches and green, the colors swirl and mix so fast that they dissolve into a white light. The words come out in a birdlike voice:

"Do you really think I will be a good mother?"

Anna looks at her mother and her mother's face is soft and open and familiar and for the second time since she came home, Anna sobs and shivers like a wet sparrow.

As adults we are capable of a much more complex understanding of the relationship between parent and child than we had as children, yet even so we oscillate between "adult" and "childish" thinking. This is especially true in relation to the woman who shaped our early years. On one hand, we see mother as an equal colleague, with whom we can talk matter-of-factly and whose feelings and opinions we understand and respect. We welcome her support in motherhood without feeling that her advice threatens our autonomy. On the other hand, at times we still see mother with a child's pair of eyes. We then hang on to her early impact on us and are convinced that whatever misdeeds she committed will greatly impact our development into motherhood. Alternatively, we may continue to see our mother through the admiring daugther's eyes, in which case our own expectations of motherhood may easily be overly sweetened.

In many ways it is a blessing that we keep the child's perspective as adults. How boring would life be if we could not bring out the child's spontaneity and playfulness, for instance? Our childishness puts magic in our lives when we just cannot stand the grimness of our adult responsibilities. Likewise, just as children do, we must believe that we are most important and that we deserve to have good things come our way. Self-enhancement is part of healthy self-esteem. Furthermore, we never outgrow our "childish" longings for hugs, comfort, and a listening ear. Finally, those of us who easily recall what it was like to be a child will have an easier time understanding our own children's thoughts and feelings. Remembering the impact and authority our parents had over us, we will strive not to misuse our power over our own children. Indeed, when we suppress and deny the continuing importance of the child we once were, we lose vital parts of ourselves.

As adult daughters, we continue to be sensitive to mother's recognition of what we do. Under the pressures of becoming a mother, we are extra vulnerable to the pulls of the original attachment. When mother takes an interest in our pregnancy and later praises us for our ways of handling our infant, we feel confident and reassured. When she criticizes our efforts or fails to empathize with our difficulties, we tend to question our abilities or may even come to dislike motherhood. Annoying as this renewed susceptibility may be, it is important to honor the emotional needs it reflects. During the emotional uproar of new motherhood we are in need of an extra allotment of attention and support. The renewed sensitivity to our childhood vision ensures that we make an effort to get these needs met.

We often become entangled in the original cord without knowing it. Blind as bats, we fail to see how our past experiences influence the present. Accordingly, we make many unhappy assumptions about our future as mothers. We may, for example, continue to believe in mother's omnipotence and our own helplessness. From this perspective, it does not make much sense to prepare for motherhood. Unconsciously, we hope to be rescued from the demands of motherhood by mother, nonetheless, who, we feel, surely will help us out as she always has. Similarily, we may continue to act as "good daughters" and instead of growing with our new responsibilities regress into a state of juvenile paralysis in which we cannot move away from mother's dictates, no matter how ill suited they may be to the present situation. When mother's approval is too important to risk losing, we will not dare to confront her with our own ideas of parenting and may find it safer to adopt her ideas of how to care for the baby.

Our continued belief in mother's dominance can mislead us in yet another way: We may come to expect that as mothers we will acquire the magic power to control what will happen to our children, just as we once thought our mothers held our future in their hands. Facing our responsibilities as mothers can be very painful because in doing so we also face our relative helplessness. While pregnant, we may at some level believe that if only we do "everything right," like making sure we get adequate food, exercise, and rest, we can assure our baby's health and safety. At the same time, the events that are beyond our control leave us in dread and we may become fixated on the possibilities of a miscarriage, a difficult labor, or an unhealthy child. Similarily, once the child is born, we will to our great dismay be reminded of the fact that we are not capable of protecting our children from every conceivable risk in life. A common expression of this struggle between the new responsibilities and the terrifying lack of power in parenthood is when the new mother feels compelled to check every ten minutes on her sleeping infant to make sure it is still breathing.

It is the new mother's task to find the right amount and kind of involvement she needs from the outside. Many new grandmothers are all too willing to jump into their old mother uniform when the baby arrives. Here is a golden opportunity to mother twofold: her own daughter and her new grandchild. As well meaning as her attempts at taking charge may be, for you the temptation is to accept mother's advice and services passively. You may dismiss your own responsibility to find out for yourself what is best for you and your baby. Your first attempts at parenting may be framed with various errors, but it is only when you take on the challenge of finding your own unique ways to parent that you will gain self-confidence as a mother.

If you know it will be difficult to withstand your mother's overly active engagement, you can do yourself a big favor by formulating and communicating clear statements of the kind of help you will want before the baby is born. It is easier to deal with hurt feelings now than when you are just home from the hospital. Tired and unaccustomed to the circumstances, you are then likely to go along with any suggestions that come your way.

The salient purpose of turning to our mothers in preparation for motherhood is to receive their blessing. The mother who can say to her daughter when she comes to her with her insecurities about becoming a mother, "You will become a good mother for your child," empowers her daughter. The daughter can give birth in confidence, whether she has her mother at her side or not. This blessing is so simple yet so laden with complex emotions that the daughter may not appreciate the emotional work involved for her mother.

THE CORD OF OUR OWN MAKING: MOTHER THROUGH THE ADULT DAUGHTER'S EYES

Anna follows Elna out to her vegetable garden. She finds a flat surface on the rock wall next to the plot where she can watch her mother work. Elna has kept a garden for as long as Anna can remember. On the first sunny day in March she takes out her trowel from the tool shed and starts turning the heavy winter soil. She stretches straight lines of string across the plot to mark her rows of plants and seeds. Small plastic flags announce what will grow in each row. As a child Anna would read the names her mother had written on the flags and imagine what spinach and corn with such beautiful names as 'Melody' spinach and 'Silver Queen' corn would look and taste like.

Today Elna weeds. She squats with her rubber boots carefully placed on each side of the green row of lettuce. Her hands work swiftly, twisting and lifting the ragweed and thistles out of the soil. Every now and then she takes a step forward. While eying the next gathering of weeds, she throws the rejected plants in the brown pail that stands next to her.

There is no trace of frustration or boredom in Elna's face. She accepts the task of weeding without a hint of resistance. In fact, Anna thinks, her mother seems to be at peace. Her movements are soft and rhythmic. Her hands and arms work in step and her legs that seem to extend deep into the earth are in keeping with the harmony of her upper body. It seems as if Elna is gently dancing a slow, earth-bound waltz.

As a teenager, Anna had often mocked her mother for her gardening mania. She could not understand how Elna could waste so much time on such a monotonous activity. Her gardening was a compulsion that prevented her mother from moving forward in life. She preferred to stay put in her strip of land rather than move into the real world and be the role model for a succesful working woman Anna so craved. "Bent over your plants," Anna had snorted, "you look like an ox strapped under the master's yoke." At this insult, Elna had let go of her usual self-control and cried into Anna's face: "How dare you ridicule my greatest passion! You have never bothered to find out what gardening means to me, have you?"

Many years have passed, but Anna still feels ashamed when she recalls this moment. At the time she had realized that she did not really know the woman who had raised her since birth. Eventually, she was able to see Elna and her special relationship to growing plants from a new perspective. In her garden, Elna is a healer. She gives of her soul to nature and nature returns liberally to her. Now, when she is close to becoming a mother, Anna sees something else. There is a sacred element in Elna's close relationship to earth. She knows how to bring up life from down under. She tends to the natural process of birth, life, death, and rebirth as if she is serving something or someone other than herself.

What we see in our mothers as adults is often radically different from the perspective we held as children. For example, when we as adult daughters reassess our mothers' impact on our lives, we can take into account the fact that their ways of parenting were affected by factors beyond their control. We are able to acknowledge that many of their concerns were neither aimed at us nor caused by us. Although knowing the reasons behind our mothers' behavior will not undo the pain they may have caused us, our adult perspective often allows us to empathize with our mothers' difficulties. A woman can, for example, see how her mother's lack of affection, which she as a child tragically perceived as a sign that she was an unlovable little girl, in reality had little to do with her, but rather with her mother's own troubles. Perhaps mother's abilities to love her child were hampered by her own experiences with a cold, rejecting mother, and she never had a chance to overcome her early injuries.

As adults, we can also understand that our mothers in many ways were products of their time and were affected by the particular expectations of what a mother should be typical of that era. Mother's unhappiness may then be attributed to her attempts to live up to the ideal of the good housewife, sacrificing her dreams of a life outside home in the process, and not, as her daughter believed, her fault. Furthermore, we can analyze our mothers' lives from a socioeconomic perspective and come to understand the cultural forces that shaped them. A mother's negligence, for example, might have been due to her financial problems that left her with little energy for her children. Likewise, a mother's low self-esteem that made her a poor role model for her daughter might be explained by the racial and sexual discrimination of her times and the restrictions it put on her life.

As painful as the awakening to a mature understanding of the mother-daughter relationship may be, it is crucial for our own transformation to mothers. When we are able to see mother as she really is, her virtues and weaknesses alike, and have compassion for her difficulties as a mother, it is no longer so difficult to accept that we also will act humane as mothers. Pent-up resentment of our own mothers' failures leaves us unsympathetic to our own mothering efforts. We run the risk of becoming our own antimothers, who promptly deliver punishment for our limitations and refuse to reward our best efforts. Humility and compassion with ourselves, and lots of them, are called for in one of the toughest jobs ever created. Without such selfrespect we will bow to the inner witch and be too humiliated to take an honest look at our parenting difficulties as we encounter them.

The kinds of questions we as adults ask about the mother-daughter bond reflect our post-Freudian way of looking at relationships and mainly concern the quality of the care we received from them: We ask what effect our mother's behavior had on us; we want to know what they did right and what they did wrong; we examine their underlying motives for their behaviors; and we wonder how their contentment and dissatisfactions with life shaped the care they gave to us. In the end, we are close to bursting with illuminating insights. But how helpful are these perceptions to our adjustment to motherhood? Are they enough to turn us into good mothers? Not by far: Comprehension of our mothers' actions may prevent us from blindly repeating the mistakes that affected us, but these insights will not necessarily make us comfortable in the mother role. We have become experts on what our children will need from us but learned nothing about what *we* need in order to mother well.

We are so well conditioned to look for flaws in our mothers that their bitterness, coldness, or despair is what we are most likely to see in them. For sure, we are rarely mistaken—as daughters we usually sense our mothers' hang-ups with uncanny accuracy—and the pain their demise caused us who were dependent on them is all too real to many of us. There is no use denying our mothers' inadequacies as it would only discourage our attempts to rise above their mistakes. Yet, hurt and sorrow cannot be all we expect to receive as daughters asking to be initiated into the mother role. Indeed, if we continue to hold on to our resentment, our refusal even to come near the original cord will immobilize us.

It is essential to keep the child's perspective if we are to empathize with and respond appropriately to our children's needs, but it is not enough. As we become new mothers it is time to use the cord of our own making and transform our youthful outlook on the mother-child relationship. Using our adult intelligence, we can turn to our mothers and learn about motherhood from the perspective of one woman giving advice to another. We relate to our mothers as women who, within the context of their times, found their particular answers to motherhood. From this perspective, we will ask radically different questions about the mother role: What does it take from a woman to mother a child? How on earth are we going to implement all our wonderful ideas on how to raise our children? *What do we need for ourselves* in order to achieve that warm and deep relationship with our daughter or son that we so wish for? Where will we find the strength to mother well?

What you find when you look to the strengths of your particular mother-daughter bond is less important—this is not a competition in who can come up with the most favorable recounting of her past. The benefits lie in the activity itself: you are looking for what makes mothering worth while, what will empower you, what will make you enjoy your child, instead of what might poison the emotional cord. Searching for the secrets in your past, you will find answers for the present. The following is an assortment of questions that women who have the opportunity might consider asking their mothers:

What does your mother remember about being a new mother?
How did motherhood change her? How did she grow? What did she have to give up?
Does she remember herself without children?
What would she do differently if she knew then what she knows now?

How did she learn to mother?
What and who helped her when the going got tough?
Who influenced her?
What did her mother tell her about motherhood?
What did she swear to do differently than her parents?

What is the biggest myth about motherhood your mother has ever heard?
If she could give you three short injunctions to help you as a new mother, what would
   they be?
What makes a good mother and why?

How did her relationship with your father change?
What improved? What went downhill?

How did you change her life?
In what ways did you challenge her?
What were the hardest part and the easiest part of raising you?
What can she tell you about motherhood that only you would appreciate?
What are the qualities you have that will help you become a good mother?

HEALING MOTHERWOUNDS

No matter how legitimate the reasons for a mother's inability to meet her daughter's needs may have been, and no matter how far away the original scenario seems now, a woman who has had inadequate mothering must *never, ever* dismiss her need for a better experience in the present. Kathie Carson, author of *In Her Image*, has this to say about the matter:

> A person who has suppressed her child's needs and viewpoint will find it almost impossible to adequately care for herself or to care about herself. Her perceptiveness and empathic concern for others may be extremely well developed; she may be a fine caretaker of everyone except herself. Championing her mother's worth at the expense of her own reflects exactly what was true in the first place: that there is no adequate *mother* in the situation. There was not in the past, and is not internally in the present.[3]

It is particularly important that we take care of our early psychological wounds as mothers. Unless a woman can acknowledge her early losses and seek help for them, these losses will cloud her fine judgments and ambitions as a mother and sap her of the emotional energy that feeds both her and her child. Her efforts may or may not have an impact on her present relationship with her mother, but they will make dramatic differences in her own life.

The internalized mother, no matter how ruthless and frightening and tricky and harmful she may be, is ours. She is in our care and she is our responsibility. We can consciously choose to transform her. We are, after all, not our mothers, and unlike our real life mothers, who may never change, *we* can learn to be different. We cannot let the inner voice of mother, which is either so critical or inept that it hinders us from becoming confident and loving mothers, have the final word.

How do you unlearn the mothering skills you once learned incorrectly? You learn with the help of others: You can volunteer at a child care center, you can visit friends whom you consider good parents, you can read parenting books, and you can take classes. You learn by seeking intimacy with other women who also are new mothers. You can also seek a healing relationship with a psychotherapist. In therapy you can look deeper into the shadow of your soul than you are able to do on your own.

It is imperative to remember that a painful past does not necessarily mean that the new mother will pass on her injuries to her child; in fact, they may be an asset to her mothering abilities. When we take up the challenge to search for our happiness despite our early losses, we will eventually develop the character that transforms us into extra sensitive and sensible mothers. As we tend to our emotional wounds, no matter how trivial they at first may seem, we will be rewarded with great wisdom that lies buried underneath the scar tissue. We will know in the deepest sense what children need from their parents.

Even if you happen to be among the fortunate women who received adequate care from your mother, you will have much to learn from women who have struggled courageously with their emotional traumas.

"Survivors of emotionally impoverished homes are forced to be scavengers, to find bits and pieces of life's essentials in all manners of places and, through their cleverness and persistence, accumulate enough to live by," says Dr. Evelyn Bassoff.[4] Regardless of the faults or fortunes of our early experiences, as new mothers we all need to search in piecemeal fashion for what we need to stay loving and giving with our children. Motherhood does not render us emotionally self-sufficient. We must assure that we are as well cared for as our infants. Just as the person healing from past injuries has learned to do, we need to look for an arsenal of caring people who can support us in different ways. Although we as adults know that no single person can fulfill all our longings, our needs are still legitimate. Unlike children, who have little say in who will provide them with what they need, we are free to choose by whom and in what way we want to be nurtured. And as mature adults, we are able to reciprocate the gifts of our benefactors in ways that fit them.

There is yet another truth about motherhood to be retrieved from the legacies of those who have overcome their pasts: Good mothering does not come effortlessly. We earn mothering with the hard work we put into the role. We must actively go searching for the care we want to give to our children and not naively assume that we will have these gifts delivered to us at the nod of a finger. We may call ourselves mothers the moment we give birth, but we learn *to mother* only by our stubborn willingness to do so.

To sum up, we have learned that attending to the pull of the emotional cord that ties us to our mothers is an important piece of work in the transformation to mother. In pregnancy, we are once again attracted to the powerful impact of our first mothering experience. In recognizing this connection, we are robbed of the illusion that our ways of mothering originate solely in our own original ideas about parenting. We come to understand that we are links in a long chain of women who are mothers. As C. G. Jung said: "Every mother contains her daughter in herself and every daughter her mother, and every woman extends backwards into her mother and forward into her daughter."[5]

Chapter 5

MOTHER CARE

In her dream, Anna wanders aimlessly among the trees of an aspen grove. The sun filters through the foliage and suggests that this is a place of great beauty and tranquility. Not so to Anna. She is anxiously searching for a path, a height, a clearing; she is not sure exactly what she expects to find. Anna comes upon a small pond. She finds a woman there, sitting on an uplifted tree root at the shoreline. She wears a mud-brown dress with long sweeping sleeves. A long heavy necklace of polished pebbles and feathers spelled off with soda-can rings and turquoise butterflies adorns her simple dress. A branch cracks under Anna's feet and the woman slowly turns her head to look at Anna. She is not surprised to see her.

Across the pond, a group of huntsmen appear. They shout and wave to catch the mysterious woman's attention.

"Dear lady, dear lady," they yell. "How can we get to you? The water is so deep and cold."

The woman gives instructions to each of them. One must carve a raft from a tree trunk, another must catch an eagle to lift him across the water, a third must wade along the shore. The huntsmen hurriedly go about their respective tasks. Anna asks the wild-natured woman if she has a command for her as well, but the woman smiles and answers that she does not. This disquiets Anna. Will the woman not be able to help her out? Why does she offer help to the witless hunters across the pond, but not to Anna? Realizing her affiliation with the wild woman, she poses another question to the woman:

"Are you a mother?"

The woman shakes her head: "I do not have any children to care for."

Meanwhile, the huntsmen have crossed the water. They greet the woman with admiring words and then fall asleep, exhausted, by the woman's feet. She begins to sing over them. It is evening. The sun is about to set behind the blue mountains. Anna quietly begins to dance to the tune of the woman's song.

In this chapter we will look at an aspect of your feminine self that you need to know by heart as a mother-to-be, new mother, any kind of mother. The matter in hand is your ability to get your own needs met as a busy mother. This is the tricky lesson of learning how to walk the narrow path of loving and caring for your child while keeping your own self in vigorous form, both when you are with and when you are away from your baby. Contrary to what you may think, you cannot live on baby love alone. As a mother you must be selfish in the sense that you must learn to care for yourself as well as you care for your offspring. If you do not give generously to yourself, you will have only crumbs left to give to your child.

As women, we are usually good at ignoring our own needs for care. We tell ourselves that we do not need anything much and that we do not deserve much of anything. Sometimes we are not even sure what needs are and whether we have them. As new mothers we are particularly careless of our right to receive succor. We fall so deeply in love with our children that we forget about ourselves, insisting that mothering is all it takes to fill our female souls.

That mothers are caring and thus do not need to have any more caring come their way is one of the biggest lies we can ever tell ourselves as new mothers. Although we may have paid attention to the suggestions on pampering ourselves in pregnancy, as soon as we become mothers we no longer find it strange that a mother can be a bottomless well of nourishment who pours out loving care to whoever thirsts for her sweet potion. A mother is no longer a woman in need: she is a self-sustained nurturer indeed. For sure, modern women know that even a mother has a right to *self-actualization*, to use her wits in other places than in her home. In fact, we believe that her only chance at happiness is to give simultaneously to society and to her family. We look with suspicion at the mother who shows signs of needing care for herself. Perhaps she has psychological difficulties, or her children are too many and too wild, or her husband is a flop. We never consider the possibility that mothers need regular maintenance to function well and not just when they show signs of distress.

Your task in pregnancy is to quiet your objections before you start believing in them and put your heart into creating the good habits you want to bring into motherhood. Hence, let us start to practice self-indulgance immediately.

PREGNANCY CARE

The next day, as she prepares her breakfast, Anna thinks about her dream. The meeting with the mysterious woman in the aspen grove lingers in her mind. The woman refuses to give Anna instructions, yet in her presence Anna's frenzied search for motherhood dissolves, and she dances a dance of liberation and gratitude. Nothing matters anymore. She just wants to dance on bare feet, hands around the baby in her body, as the sky glows in bright evening colors.

The dream indicates to Anna that the intense period in which she has been hunting for answers to her questions and doubts is coming to an end. What has she learned? The specifics seem irrelevant to her transformation. The huntsmen have accomplished their mission. Fatigued from the effort, the carriers of her mind's quest for comprehension fall asleep at the wise woman's feet.

The woman who knows more than she will say does not need to tell Anna what to do. In her presence, Anna recovers acceptance. Her joy finds expression in the unbidden movements of her dance.

Anna measures the tea leaves into the teapot. She pours the boiling water over the black leaves and watches them swirl with the spinning water current. She places the lid over the rising steam. Then she cuts two thick slices of crusty bread, butters them, and puts a slice of cheese on one piece of bread and a glaze of honey on the other. She remembers the decorated plate her mother once brought back from Yorkshire, a romantic scene from a country fox hunt painted on it, and finds the plate at the top shelf of the kitchen cupboard. She carries the plate with the two sandwiches and the teapot into the study. She will eat by the bay window today.

Anna sits down to eat her breakfast. Why is it so difficult to arrive at the very simple? she wonders. Simplicity is only experienced after one surrenders to the incomprehensible. Anna sips her tea.

The secret to becoming a mother who feels alive and content in caring for her child, as opposed to an exhausted and discontented mother, lies in a woman's ability to stay connected to her self. She knows her own needs and desires and takes measures to assure their fulfillment. She is a woman who knows herself; she knows when to seek solace and when to call for company. She is not afraid to ask for help as needed, yet is confident enough to blaze her own trails when her convictions command. She listens carefully to advice, then throws it into her inner waters to see whether it will float or sink. Advice that does not survive this test is not worth keeping. She is a woman with good instincts. She keeps herself out of trouble by following her inspirations about what direction, position, and action will best protect her.

How does she sustain her sense of self? By cherishing who she is. She soothes and nourishes the self that has run dry. She talks sense into herself: "I am important. I am loved. I deserve care." She retreats to restore her inner resources and she will not return until she has found her manna and is ready for her relationships and projects again. Since she knows how to protect herself, she can allow herself to be open to other people in mind and spirit. She trusts that in sharing herself she will not allow herself to be neglected. Herself well taken care of, she can be fully present with her child.

If you want to learn how to stay connected to yourself in the face of motherhood you must be prepared to practice. Your baby may take your work for granted, but you should not take yourself for granted. Mothering requires excellent cooking skills. You must know your ingredients well, know where to get them and how to prepare them. You must develop a feel for what goes into the pot, add a little of this and a little of that, then stir, whisk, and taste to your liking. When it is time to eat, remember to set a plate for yourself, and as you dish out your nourishment, be proud and grateful for what you have accomplished. By cooking for others you learn to estimate your own resources; you know that when the pot is empty it is empty and there is nothing for anyone, and when times are good there is enough for everyone and for guests. It makes no sense to blame meagreness on your lack of time and money, on your husband, or on your work. You can prepare a satisfying meal out of a pile of rocks if you know how to care for yourself. Mothering is a skill built on determination and good faith. Add a good measure of guts, spunk, and grits and you are cooking.

PREGNANCY AND THE PECULIAR

Anna has only one thing on her mind: black, salty, licorice fish—the candy you will find in the Scandinavian shop in Aunt Ellen's Minnesota and nowhere else. Anna cannot get these licorice fish out of her mind. Her mouth begins to water as she imagines sticking the candy between her lips. Simultaneously salty and sweet tasting, they challenge your taste buds to identify the unlikely combination of flavors. Chewing the candy is like gulping a mouthful of ocean water, and you will cough and spit until you have rid yourself of the scare. It is better to let the fish rest on your tongue and let it slowly melt into a tasteful blend of opposites.

These heavenly treats are nowhere to be found. Anna has visited every gourmet department and specialty store in town in a desperate attempt to track down her sweet taste memory. She even bought some sweet licorice and rolled the pieces in salt, but they turned out to be a poor duplicate. She craves Real Black Licorice Fish, the original childhood experience.

Perhaps she can contact the nursing home where poor senile Aunt Ellen now resides and get then to look up the name of the little Scandinavian store? Under favorable circumstances, the candy will be mailed to her within a week. It seems like a long time, but she is prepared to wait for the fulfillment of her most pressing desire.

It has long been noted that pregnant women acquire strange tastes. Ice cream out of the carton, pickles with extra salt, and pumpkin pie in July are considered typical edibles. When you first become pregnant, you are warned to expect the most bizarre behavior to satisfy your new appetites. As a pregnant woman you will go to any length under any circumstances to satisfy your cravings. These characteristics can be successfully applied to your emotional needs in pregnancy as well. Do not be surprised if your preferences are nothing like what used to interest you before. A woman with a fat belly needs different enjoyments than her skinny sisters need.

In general, women seem to turn to more low-key, "basic" activities during pregnancy, intending to create more rest and less stress in their lives. This may require that you make a written list of your commitments, and if the list measures more than the length of your arm, it will be necessary to weed out the undertakings you can do without. Solitude is often a new priority that comes with the introvertive state of pregnancy. A quiet evening in the armchair, an aimless stroll after work, a weekend spent where sky and horizon meet are activities that seem far more satisfying than finding out what Liz thinks of Lou. Herein lies the difference between frustration and satisfaction with your nine months of childbearing: either you go on as if nothing unusual is happening or you realize that your new adventure requires a new strategy, after which you set out to discover what is asked of you.

If you are supposed to have peculiarities in pregnancy, why not prove yourself peculiar beyond all expectations? Allow yourself to seek the perfect peach, the exact word to describe your feelings, and the right piece of music to fit your mood. Find the most relaxing position in the most comfortable chair, and the perfect dress to go with your pregnant beauty. Do not be lax about yourself. It is worth the effort to search for your own well-being, because selflove translates into love for your child.

In pregnancy, your old methods for staying sane and functioning may no longer work. All of a sudden your childless friends do not seem to have any empathy with your feelings. To find true understanding you prefer to seek out the company of those who also have parenting on their mind. A new circle of acquaintances evolves. You may also need to modify the ways in which you give to yourself. The thrill of downhill skiing or bareback galloping is no longer a safe release of tension. There is no other way out but to resort to less challenging physical activities that better fit your new status. Similarly, when the creative flow that previously urged you to produce short stories, quilts, or gourmet meals temporarily shuts down, you are impelled to find other creative outlets.

After pregnancy is completed and motherhood begins, you can expect to make yet new adaptations. There is no longer a physical barrier to prevent you from returning to your prepregnancy activities, but there may well be a psychological one. In becoming a mother you have changed in spirit. You have a different view of yourself and of your place in the world, and thus new demands emerge. Consequently, you must again use your creativity to find new ways to nurture yourself.

PREGNANCY AND CREATIVITY

As with all creative acts, pregnancy holds the power to transform the turmoil of your inner life into something profusely meaningful. The means—writing, painting, singing, dancing, or doing nothing at all but keeping your senses open—could not be less important. The one condition you must meet to get to the sum and substance of your transformation is to be honestly willing to immerse yourself in the process. Your open senses allow you to note your corpulent bulkiness and the small blue vessels on your belly, your inner torrents of excitement and moments in the blue, and the verbal good-wishes and silent flickers of jealousy of others. All and everything knit together into the tapestry of pregnancy. It is your task to give a unique meaning to what you have collected.

Creative activities help you gain mastery: Write down your thoughts, paint your feelings, dance out the movements in your belly, and you will find that instead of being a vessel passively carrying human creation, you are now the agent of the creative process. You have control over the spectacle within your body. Only you know the details of the drama and the impact the transformation has on those who are involved. You are documenting a part of your life sui generis. This creation is truly yours to grow and mature from.

Your creative acts will also help you approach the parts of your experiences of pregnancy that frighten you: The wild woman lurking inside—who is she and why is she insisting on being present? The wolf, the lioness, the stranded whale—what do they have to tell about motherhood? Through simple creations you can express what you are just starting to know but are not yet ready to integrate into your being. Roars, growls, and soft syllables on a string; rocking movements and the squatting position; "don't-you-dare-touch-him" and "I have never felt such magnificence"—all can be explored and practiced for those who dare to imagine.

THE NESTING INSTINCT

Eight months pregnant, Anna breaks through her resistance to making any kinds of practical preparations for Miriam. Up to now Anna has been afraid to set her hands on anything that would signify her confidence in the future, as if attending to practical matters would challenge fate to turn against her. Gathering baby items was serious risk taking, she had felt. How could she be so sure there would be a baby to wear the baby clothes and to sleep in the crib? What if she lost the baby in childbirth?

Now Anna is making up for lost time. She paints the walls of the nursery in two mild colors while Thomas sews and hangs the curtains. She scours the floor until the sparkling finish reflects the baby furniture and then scans the second-hand stores for a small rug that will match the colors of the room. With Thomas's assistance, she spends an entire evening putting together the wooden cradle Baby Thomas once was rocked to sleep in. Anna layers the cradle with white linen and the baby quilt her mother already has presented them with. Finally she drags the heavy chest of drawers from the study into the nursery. She cannot wait until she can fill the drawers with baby clothes.

The "nesting instinct"—the home-based cleaning, designing, and rearranging typical of late pregnancy—is a way to rid yourself of some nervousness on the eve of delivery. These creative activities are also simple welcoming rites for the child. They are a way of mentally bringing the child in your body into the world, of saying, "Yes, I am now as ready as I can be to welcome you into my life." Preparing a nursery, looking at baby clothes, and sewing a baby blanket are acts that signal the imminence of delivery: A child will soon be born who will rearrange the innermost chambers of your life.

As many pregnant women have commented, even the most mundane chores suddenly seem utterly meaningful to them. Hands-on work, such as folding clothes, ironing, knitting, and sewing, function as emotional outlets for the pressure building internally. The energy flows through the same hands that soon will hold the child. Busy hands can be soothing, gentle, sensitive—a first expression of love toward the child. Life is in your hands.

PLAYTIME

When else should there be ample time for play and laughter if not in pregnancy? A good belly laugh sends rolling waves through the uterine water. Play creates ripples of contentment in the torso. Skip and jump with the grace of an elephant, drop your chin in awe, breathe in the fresh scent of a newborn day, whistle your favorite melody—there are plenty of ways to bring out your playfulness. The little girl you once were is not far away; you can, if you spend some time on it, reexperience her delights. An afternoon in the toy store, a return to her favorite fairy tales, or a mouthful of chocolate pudding on the palate and you have evoked her presence.

When we play, we are not concerned with acting appropriately or accomplishing what must be done. We are present in the moment. We do things because they make us feel good right now. Our wildest fantasies and most splendid imaginings become tailored to satisfy just the kind of persons we are. The little girl we carry within will let us know what she likes and dislikes in life. She will show us the way to magic:

> The Inner Child consists of all our childlike feelings, instincts, intuitions, spontaneity, and vitality. It is naturally open and trusting unless it learns to shut down for self-protection. It is emotional and expressive until condemned for being what it is-a child. It is playful until it is crushed for being childish. This Inner Child is creative until ridiculed for its expression. It is magical until it is punished for using its imagination. We can bury it, distort it, handicap it, make it sick, but we can't get rid of it.[1]

KINSHIP

So here she is, finally: at her own baby shower. How she has anticipated this moment. Next to giving birth, this is the event of pregnancy she has surrounded with the greatest mystique. She has mocked the modern rite for its pink and blue romanticism (the mother-to-be is expected to appear ecstatic over teddy bears and miniature baby shoes), the implicit sex-role stereotyping (who has ever heard about a shower for the father-to-be?), and its superficiality (the ohs and ahs she is expected to produce during the highlight of the evening—the gift-opening ceremony). Yet, she also recognized the event as a happy occasion in which she could share her mounting excitement over the baby with her friends. The closer she got to birth, the more she had looked forward to this particular evening.

The room is full of chatter and laughter. Anna sits propped up in an armchair while the other women gather around her. Her friends do not spare her; comments about her ponderous size and flustered appearance never seem to bore them, they tease her about her infinite self-doubts, and they predict how ridiculously amateurish she will act as a new mother. Anna admits to herself that despite her cynicism about the intrinsic value of baby showers, she is truly enjoying herself. Her friends are wonderful, and here they are all gathered together to celebrate with her. Anna is smitten with excitement: SHE is having a baby, SHE has made it through pregnancy, SHE is close to birth. At this moment, pregnancy is the most important experience she has had in her life. May her exhilaration not precipitate an early labor, she adds to temper her self-inflation.

The celebration reminds her of her wedding. Then why is Thomas not here? Does he belong here or not? She has mixed feelings. She wishes there would be a social event to commemorate their joint commitment to the baby, yet if this had been a party with both men and women, the unique womanesque atmosphere would be lost. Selfishly, she would miss her friends' acknowledgment of her personal accomplishment in pregnancy and their affirmation of her uniqueness as a woman, which the baby shower attends to. She likes being praised, indulged, envied, and celebrated! In her friends' presence, it suddenly is easy for her to accept her new identity as an (almost) mother, which she has struggled with on her own for so many months.

Her friends will not let her withdraw into her own quiet thoughts for long. They want to know what names she has selected for the baby, the worst and the best of being pregnant, what happened in the Lamaze classes, and what plans she has made for birth. Later, the childbirth stories come out. Everyone, mother or not, has one to tell. The pain and the danger are left unspoken for her sake but linger there anyway. Then, quickly they turn back to safer ground, and her friends commence their assigned task of bolstering her confidence: They are certain that with Anna's constitution, she will pop out the baby in no time, they predict Anna's bravery and Thomas's feebleness, and they paint a beautiful scene of a newborn baby gazing into Anna's teary eyes. And their pep talk works: Anna feels ready to proceed right to the delivery room.

In the past, the extended family and neighbors came together to share in all the major life transitions of their members from cradle to grave. The well-being of the individual was a concern to everyone. Childbirth was a social act as important to society as its leadership or social order. The very survival of the village or the farm depended on the reproductive stamina of its workforce. Sheila Kitzinger describes how pregnancy and childbirth operate within a cultural context of customs and rituals:

> Birth is a keypoint in the social system. When a baby is expected the pregnant woman is one of the major protagonists in a process of social integration which unites previously disparate elements and reinforces weak links in the chain of interaction. The bringing of a child to life is not just a personal, private act, but one which actively promotes social cohesion.[2]

In our society, which is structured around the small and private unit of the nuclear family, we have almost forgotten how important it is for the primigravida to be surrounded by others who can help her pass through the transformation feeling safe and valued. In lieu of the extended family, many of must construct our own support system with the help of friends and neighbors. As men and women join to share the parental responsibilities, new customs around childbirth emerge. Many women see their husbands as their most intimate relation and source of emotional support in pregnancy. The involvement of the husband solidifies their being in the creation together and prepares them jointly for the birth of their child.

Pregnancy is also an activity which creates social cohesion among *women* themselves. Our mates deserve all due respect, but they do not take care of women's need to get together and tell their own kind of stories. Childbirth brings women together around an act that encapsulates much of what it means to be a woman. Women get together to word about maternal feelings, the implications of one's biological nature, sexism, sexuality, aging, and whatever else can be studied in the new mother. It is a social event that brings women together around the recondite propensities of life.

In the preparations for motherhood we can all partake. We can offer words of wisdom. We can cause a stir with our childbirth stories, break clean with a good joke, and recite poetry until every eye is watering. Some of us can give a comprehensible explanation of the neuromuscular mechanisms behind uterine contractions. Others will make baby clothes and cook delicious meals. Yet others will add a political, feminist, historical, spiritual, or purely personal perspective of women's propensities for childbearing.

Pregnancy concerns all women. We are either little girls wondering how babies are made, teenagers looking at our future, career women finding solace in the noncompetitive atmosphere of childbirth, middle-aged women reminiscing, or old ladies readying ourselves to leave off for the next generation. Regardless of her own age, a woman can look to the pregnant woman and find vital aspects of womanhood present. She will find abundant evidence of female strength and endurance. She can ponder the bravery of women, study their capacity to love and care, and see sensitivity and emotionality put to good use. Further, she can see what fierce commitment looks like and she can marvel over women's physical strength and psychological power. The attention she receives does wonders for the pregnant woman at the epicenter of the commotion.

WOMEN OF YOUR OWN KIND

People share in your transformation in many different ways. Your husband participates as your equal in the preparations for birth, your mother provides you with trust and wisdom and a sense of history, your friends give nurturance and encouragement. Women of your own kind, that is, other mothers-to-be and new mothers, have another advantage: With them you can be as obsessed with baby matters as you wish and this without apology.

People who truly understand what you are describing about pregnancy are hard to come by. Becoming a mother for the first time is a one-time event in a woman's life that catches her full involvement when she is going through the process but then falls pray to forgetfulness. By the time her child is a toddler she wonders to herself what the big deal about becoming a mother was. She may have more children, but she will never go through the initial transformation again. By the time she becomes a grandmother she no longer remembers the thoughts and feelings motherhood once gave rise to. Nor are our partners always our best source of understanding. The transformation to father has its own course. Hence, in order to find true empathy with the events of your first pregnancy, you are better off seeking your like.

Women meet at childbirth classes, at the hospital bed, at La Leche league meetings, at the playground, or in the diaper aisle. These meetings, informal or structured, connect women and give them an experience of *community*: of belonging to a context in which you are recognized as a valued member. Seeing yourself reflected in others, you can make sense of your own thoughts and feelings. This is a safe place in which to vent your frustrations and laugh at your lapses. Shared laughter and pain turn the extraordinary into the ordinary and the ordinary into the extraordinary.

THE MATRON

Many European countries have a tradition of midwifery as their preferred way to take care of a woman's childbirth needs. The midwife is traditionally concerned with both a safe delivery and the expectant mother's psychological well-being. She is attentive to the woman's emotional needs and helps her through pregnancy and delivery with a mixture of practical advice and emotional support. Sheila Kitzinger describes the midwife as the "shepherdess" of birth who shepherds mother and child through delivery and the early postpartum days.[3] Modern-time hospitals try to create a similar environment with homelike delivery rooms, educational classes to prepare the new parents, and skillful nursing during the hospital stay. Through these measures the new mother is well taken care of in pregnancy and birth. However, after she leaves the hospital, the system seems to abandon her abruptly. As she enters the quiet atmosphere of her living quarters, the door slams shut behind her. There is no one to bother her, no one to supervise her moves. She is alone with her baby, at last. It is time to be a family: mother, father, child. How she has waited for this moment! Then again, after a while she begins to wonder, Who is there to help her out? Whom can she ask? It is so quiet around the house. It is time to summon her *matron*.

As new mothers we need large volumes of loving support from women who are seasoned in baby matters. It is nice to have someone at hand who knows the remedy to breast engorgement and can suggest fifty ways to calm an upset baby, and who can think up a feast from the last cans of tuna and corn in the kitchen. Moreover, we need support beyond practicalities. We need someone who understands what new motherhood does to a woman's mind, who can listen acceptingly to our mixed reviews of mother bliss, and who has a full appreciation of the hard labor that resumes after birth. We need someone who can keep track of us when we get lost in the deep seas of our infants' eyes, who can remind us to eat and rest and shower and whatever else we forget in our preoccupation with the baby. In short, as new mothers we need the support from those who can truly see to us and our needs.

Whether for practical or for psychological reasons, few women of our times will engage their mothers for this job. Yet, little is won when we ignore the importance of our mothers to our lives, because along with them goes our awareness of our need for support and guidance. We are much better off acknowledging that the help our mothers symbolize is essential, and then seeking out this support whether it be from our mothers or from other women. It does not matter whom we choose, as long as we remember the concept of motherly care and why we need such care as we make our arrangements for upcoming events.

Your mother, or any other experienced woman you choose as your matron, can add the seasoned perspective you lack. She sees baby's resilience when you can see only his fragility; she can soothe when you worry; and she can remind you of your humanity when you are too hard on yourself. If she is very wise indeed, she will know when to keep her lips sealed and let you find your own way, and when to extend a helping hand and let you watch and learn. But guiding you into the mother role is ideally not all your matron will do for you. She will also know to nurture you, because she thinks that you are deserving of some extra attention as a new mom. If this description sounds too much like the Ideal Mother you just have learned not to believe in, so be it. Just remember that new mothers are not as freewheeling as you might think: you will need this kind of caring help.

AFTER BIRTH: CARING FOR OURSELVES AS NEW MOTHERS

No matter how liberated and independent and strongwilled we consider ourselves as women, in motherhood many of us nevertheless question the right to time away from our children: Your baby, so tiny and helpless, how could you possible leave him? You love him so, you spend so much time admiring him, nursing him, comforting him—you understand his needs better than anyone else. You can feel into the marrow of your bones how important you are to him. Your strong identification with your baby's situation is good evidence that you have established the necessary emotional attachment to your child.

As mothers, we do not come first anymore. Our children do. There are no bones about it. We can postpone our needs; they cannot. We know how to wait; they know only the moment. We can find numerous ways to bring pleasure to ourselves; their pleasures center around physical comfort and human contact. You do not need a degree in psychology to realize that neglecting the immediate needs of an infant has far more severe consequences for the child than it does for the adult. As parents we carry the responsibility for the child dependent on our care and we must attend to their immediate demands. Yet, ignoring ourselves readily becomes a habit. A year down the road we are still only intent on our children's needs. Years later we do not even remember what we need and like for ourselves.

When you can acknowledge your natural limitations as a mother and realize that you cannot be everything to your children, you can take actions to ensure that they get their complete allowance of emotional care in other ways. Let other people have a chance to know your child. Dad is the mandatory candidate, but there are others, such as grandparents, neighbors and friends, who may be able to give to your child what mom yet has to work on. The people to whom you can entrust your child will enrich your child's life in ways uniquely theirs. Meanwhile, you are given a chance to retreat for a while and regain your enthusiasm for the mother role.

In real life, our ability to give to others fluctuates. Some days we can give more, some days less. This is the natural ebb and flow of our emotional lives. Yet most of us have trouble accepting our limitations as nurturers. We love our children so much and we want to give them our full hearts, incessantly, unambivalently. It is extremely painful to recognize the occasions when we fail our children. We are well aware of how much our children need us to encourage their adventures and to affirm their being. We know the pain a mother who withdraws her attention can inflict upon her child, as well as how frightening a mother who has lost her temper is. Few can pass up the guilt feelings and selfreproach that follow after we, inevitably, find ourselves guilty on any of these accounts. These negative feelings build internal dykes which the fresh waves of psychic restoration cannot penetrate.

Instead of telling yourself that you are a failure as a mother when you are weary, congratulate yourself for being so alert as to realize your condition, and then do something about the sad situation: Do you need time off? When did you last get acknowledgment for the work you do? Have you had enough rest, laughter, irresponsibility? How about a dinner for two? In due time, you will find your own remedies. The sooner you start your inquiries into the matter, the better.

When you stay open and alive in spirit you can take in the natural vitality of your child. Your heart warms, your eyes brighten, your face relaxes—you are in love with your child. You are open to his full range of feelings. You see what the child is seeing, you hear what he is hearing. To give to him is to give to yourself. But if you are locked inside yourself, you will not be able to take in what your child has to offer. The vitality of your child may register, but it will not feed your spirit.

If you think that your child can give you a sense of aliveness, you are kidding yourself. Rather, by taking responsibility for your own well-being, you will remain open to the joys of your baby. The child drinks greedily from your well, but you cannot quench your thirst in his rivulets.

WHICH ARE MORE IMPORTANT: YOUR CHILD'S NEEDS OR YOUR OWN?

After birth, you will be put in many thorny situations that will test your judgment in balancing your needs versus your child's. What will you do in a situation like this one? Your infant is sleeping contentedly by your side at night, but you are listening to all his little rumblings and whimpers and cannot fall asleep yourself. What do you do now? Should you put your child back into his crib? If you decide to separate the two of you, should this crib be by your bedside or in a different part of the house? How important is physical closeness to his developing sense of trust? What is more important, your need for sleep or his need for human contact? Is there a way you can have both? Or picture yourself in this situation: Numerous studies show the benefits of breast-feeding, but you simply do not care for it. Your breasts are heavy and sore, you sit stiff as a board through the feedings, and your child fusses as he senses your nervousness. If you have tried the nurse's instructions, La Leche league information, and every book written on breast-feeding and you still cannot get the hang of it, what will you do? Will you endure for your child's sake or let your baby take to the bottle, hoping the advocates of breast-feeding are wrong? What option will promote the best contact between the two of you? Is it more important to honor your own feelings than to take what is believed to be the best alternative for your child?

To convince yourself that you are right when others cry "wrong" takes a good deal of self-confidence. It is much easier to follow the advice of those who claim to know what is best for your infant. You genuinely want to do everything in your power to bring up your child happily, and if you are given convincing arguments for a particular approach to mothering, you will of course want to follow this advice. The problem with adopting standards set by others, however, is that they consistently lead you away from yourself and your own feelings. When you repeatedly abandon your own perceptions, you start to mistrust yourself. Your instinctual sense of what you must do to find your own well-being is jeopardized.

True self-confidence springs forth when you act in accordance with your own feelings and your own beliefs. Your sense of self—your well-being—matters more than anything to your child. He is finely attuned to your state of mind: with the sensitivity of a compass needle he will pick up your frustrations and anxiety, and in his body he will feel your tensions and your numbness. When you choose to ignore your own feelings, you are in effect teaching your child that violating the boundaries that protect your well-being, his or yours, is an acceptable choice.

The best you can do as a new parent is to know yourself, and to trust that by following your intuitions for what you need and want, you will also recognize what to give to your child. Sheila Kitzinger puts the idea this way:

> It is not just a matter of a mother performing an action, such as suckling an infant, but also of how she *feels* about what she does. And whether or not [the mother] behaves in an easy, spontaneous and above all non-anxious manner may be a good deal more important than the system of child-rearing she adopts or the fact that she holds or does not hold the child, or even that she breast- or bottle-feeds it.[4]

No matter what choices you make to see your child through his infancy—and there are rarely clear-cut answers—when your feelings are at odds with what is recommended for infants you must always make sure to include both of you, and not, as tradition dictates, to sacrifice yourself to your child. Your child's awareness of himself, which at first is united with your sense of self, is simultaneously wounded.

Added to the advice you have received on how best to meet your child's needs, you will now have another set of expectations against which to measure your adequateness as a mother: whether you are in possession of healthy feelings about yourself or not. In comparison to other instructions available to the new mother, this may be the most disturbing idea of all. The emphasis on the relation of your inner satisfaction to your child's well-being threatens your already shaky self-confidence by targeting the very core of who you are. Not only must you follow the current trend to give natural birth to your baby and breast-feed him in order to be considered a good mother: If you are not psychologically in tiptop shape, you are now told that you will negatively affect your child's development with your poor self-image. Another burdensome responsibility is lain upon your shoulders. This time you are asked to be happy, no matter how hard the transformation to mother may have hit you.

Truthfully, few of us enjoy a stable, tranquil sense of self at the time of our first childbirth. It cannot be overemphasized that the transformation to mother is a time of inner turmoil. As a new mother, you need to remind yourself constantly of how demanding becoming a mother is. Give yourself plenty of leeway and compassion when you find yourself functioning well below your optimum. Keep these three principles in mind: (1) *Account for your own lowpoints*. It is natural to have them. Do not let fantasies of becoming the Ideal Mother seduce you. (2) *Compensate for your insufficiencies*. Find help and support from others when you need to. (3) *Stay with yourself*. The more conscious you are of yourself and how you relate to your child, the more opportunity there is for growth for you.

Chapter 6

A MOTHER'S BODY

When the Body Speaks

If you want to know me,
waste no time to guess from my actions.
All you have to do is come a little closer.
My body will tell you who I am.

See the oval shadow my body casts on the ground,
a cloak covering both my past and my future,
shading the little girl I once was,
and my child who will soon open her eyes
to the brightness of the first day of her life.

See my generous bosom,
I am ready to give of myself.
I will put my child close to me,
fill her with my milk and warmth
and the fragrance of my body
until she rests full and content in my arms.

I stand square on the ground,
like a seaman on a rolling ship,
ready to absorb every pounding wave
and let the water of life rinse over me,
showering me with courage and vigor.

I have invited life to share my space.
See how full I am with love,
a magical goodness that grows inside.

Self-respect lives in the waters of my womb,
enough to carry both me and you,
reaching out to all tender life of the planet.

Finally look me in the eyes
and see the excitement twinkle blue;
the deep blue color of infinite possibilities.
I meet your stare with confidence,
because I am bringing life to you.

The single most influential ingredient to facilitate a woman's psychological transformation to mother is the unique physicality of pregnancy. The pregnant body prepares a woman for motherhood in many creative ways. First, the body connects the pregnant woman to her inner self. The body candidly reflects the many changes in the self that take place in pregnancy. A woman can see and feel in her body how she is changing from month to month. Second, the body connects her to the power of her feminine self. It instinctively knows how to mother the child and is thus a fine source of confidence for the new mother. Last but not least, the body connects the pregnant woman to her child. Starting with the quickening, the woman can feel her child's presence in her body.

In this chapter we will examine the pregnant body from these three perspectives of self-knowledge, femininity, and the relationship to the child. The intention is to show how the practice of body awareness will bring the pregnant woman closer to her mother-self.

THE BODY CONNECTS THE PREGNANT WOMAN TO HER INNER SELF

Starting at conception, it is in the depths of your body that all is happening: The fertilized egg travels through the fallopian tube and attaches itself to the surface of the endometrium. Multiplying cells rapidly form every organ of the developing fetus. The wall of the uterus thickens and fills with amniotic fluid to protect the fetus. There is a busy exchange of nutrients and oxygen through the nourishing placenta. From the very beginning of pregnancy, your body is engaged in the tasks of holding, nurturing, and protecting the new life placed in its care.

Your body is your inner mother, the source and ground of your mothering activities. When you are intimately in tune with its workings, your body will guide you in caring for your child, both in pregnancy and after birth. Reliable, honest, and always present, your body will tell you what you need to know. It will provide you with a form of knowledge you cannot expect to find in books, a wisdom innate in your being.

In order to understand the wisdom of the body, we must learn to interpret its unique language. *Body awareness* is not only a matter of understanding the physiological process of gestation. The concept also relates to our understanding of the relationship between body and psyche. In our culture, we commonly consider our mind to be the natural center of self-awareness. We do not think of the areas below the neckline as a source of information about ourselves. Yet our bodies tell a different truth about us. The way we move, breathe, and carry ourselves reflects our primal, instinctive selves that our socialized minds may not register. In Jungian psychology, it is said that the body is our link to the unconscious.

Jungian psychoanalyst Marion Woodman clearly understands the importance of the body for self-knowledge when she discusses how both the body and the dream relate to the unconscious:

> Body movements, I realized, can be understood as a walking dream. In its spontaneous movements the body is like an infant crying out to be heard, understood, responded to, much as a dream is sending out signals from the unconscious. . . . The body is the unconscious in its most immediate and continuous form; the dream is also the unconscious, though as a body of images it lacks both the immediacy and continuity of the physical body.[1]

Our bodies, like our dreams, are tools with which we gain access to the realms of our psyches we otherwise would not be in touch with. Our bodies complement our rational minds and provide us with an expanded vision of ourselves.

Alexander Lowen, the founder of the bioenergetic approach to body-oriented psychotherapy, agrees that the body and its feelings are loyal to sources of the personality that are much deeper than the roots of reason. He says:

> In a healthy person the irrational is not suppressed in favor of the reasonable. The healthy person accepts his feelings even when they run counter to the apparent logic of the situation. . . . The body is abandoned when the irrational is denied and feeling is repressed. To reclaim the body, an individual must accept the irrational within himself.[2]

Alexander Lowen compares the fear so many of us have of our instinctual bodies with the fear we may have of an animal:

> On the body level, the human being is an animal whose behavior is unpredictable from a rational point of view. This doesn't mean that the body or the animal is dangerous, destructive, and uncontrollable. The body and the animal obey certain laws, which are not the laws of logic. The animal lover finds the animal perfectly comprehensible. To the person in touch with his body, the feelings of the body make complete sense.[3]

Sadly enough, many of us have learned to ignore communication from our bodies. From an early age we are taught to hold back our feelings; to "keep a stiff upper lip," to "swallow the bitter medicine," and to "hold our heads high." Without hesitation, we override signals of hunger, sleepiness, or need for movement if doing so will satisfy some desire the ego finds more important. We may accurately read the body language of others but not pay the slightest attention to our own reactions. Few of us trust our "gut feeling." Expecting our bodily instincts to be embarrassing rather than helpful, we carefully try to control them so that they not reveal more to us than we wish to know.

We, adults of the nineties, are often so particular about our bodies, shaping and reshaping them as if we were sculpturing precious figurines, that it would seem that body awareness is our number one priority. We find the willpower to go on liquid diets, push ourselves through strenuous workouts, and even use plastic surgery to perfect our exteriors. The emphasis we place on health and appearance may give the impression that we know our bodies well. In reality, this relationship is only skin-deep. Our efforts concern how we can make our physique fit the image we would like to project of ourselves rather than what we are truly like.

We can witness this physioemotional injury in the woman who battles against her growing body with diets and exercise in pregnancy. The woman does not trust the goodness of her maternal body. For her, the changing body is a frightening sign that a destructive *witch mother* is about to take over.[4]

In a positive way, the body can be likened to a cathedral, a magnificent physical structure designed to hold the human spirit. The body draws the viewer's attention to certain characteristics that are essential to the personality. It also protects the self and will hide or distort as readily as it will reveal the innermost truths about a person. In the course of time, the body is a testament to how we have lived. Erect or collapsed, open or ironclad, it discloses what the occupant has experienced in life.

The mind must establish a close relationship to its physical structure. If we never consciously take possession of our bodies, the treasures of wisdom they contain will be lost. We need to enter the temples of our souls respectfully and closely observe what is laid open to us. When we learn to respect the truth of our bodies, our physical selves and mental selves can move in synchrony. Our vitality comes forth. We can take in life and give back to life with the richness of all our senses.

THE PREGNANT BODY PREPARES A WOMAN FOR MOTHERHOOD

Anna spends extra time in front of the mirror these days. She examines her waistline, her heavy breasts with their dark brown areolas, her blotchy face. She deliberates about her gestures and practices her movements. While she scrutinizes herself in the mirror, she cannot help but notice: She has a new body. This new body in the mirror lets her clearly see what she has been struggling to formulate in her mind: Who is she? Who is she becoming?

"I am draped in a beautiful veil," Anna thinks to herself. It is as if she once again stands as a bride. This time, however, she is without a white gown. Only the long veil that falls in sweeping layers from the crown of her head covers her pregnant body. She examines the garment carefully. It is made of tan-colored lace so delicate the light will even shine through the edges embroidered with grapeleaves and birds. This revealing outfit she will wear until the end of her pregnancy. She knows of no other way to keep away from others what is becoming more and more apparent: She is naked under her veil. The transparent veil exposes her to others, and at the same time she is exposed to them. Stares, comments, appraisal, even the touch of a stranger's hand penetrate her veil.

Her mission is to look deep into the mirror and with attentive, searching eyes look for answers. After she finds confirmation she will shed her veil of pregnancy and it will fall to the ground and reveal the woman person who has been hiding underneath.

In pregnancy, as your focus of attention shifts from the outside world to the inside, you are offered an excellent opportunity to develop awareness of your body. The signs are subtle at first, like the tenderness in your breasts, a tingling bladder, or your new appetite. Soon, however, the subtlety is gone. Every part of the body seems involved in the process of creating new life. Although the degree of physiological and hormonal change is highly variable between women, many symptoms are common. Skin pigmentation darkens in the face, abdominal wall, and genitals. The sweat glands are frequently hyperactive. Acidic secretions from the stomach are pushed into the lower esophagus and can cause heartburn. Bloating and constipation are also common, and pressure on the lower intestines can result in hemorrhoids. Breathing is modified. The diaphragm lifts as the growing uterus exerts pressure and there is an increase in the volume of air breathed each minute. The breasts show superficial veins, the areolas grow and pigment, and colostrum may leak from the nipple. All in all, you can expect a thorough refresher course on the anatomy and physiology of the body.

The extensive physical changes of pregnancy have corresponding psychological effects on the pregnant woman. She is made aware of the raw, uninhibited force with which her body expresses itself, no matter how hard she consciously tries to resist. She no longer seems to be in charge of either body or mind. This experience can be rather disturbing, depending on how unfamiliar her wild, uncanny side is to her.

"Pregnancy brings out the self we usually are not aware of," says Lena Reagan, a certified massage therapist (CMT) in Boulder, Colorado. She believes that the lower part of our bodies is the center of our female selves. In here reside the deepest, most carefully protected parts of our being: our rage and aggression, our sexuality, our vulnerable core. When the growing fetus fills out the womb it is as if there is no space left to hold in the powerful emotions of the deep self. Feelings and thoughts we normally would keep to ourselves are pushed up and out in the open. Repressed anger at certain people or circumstances, revived sadness over past losses, or even a sense of childish joy and impishness that is uncharacteristic of a person may surface.

Although pregnancy certainly can bring a woman into closer touch with her body, it is also common for the opposite to happen. Since most of us are not used to being in such close contact with our bodily selves, it can be a shock to receive the stimuli from our wide-open senses. We wonder whether there perhaps is something wrong with us. Feeling ashamed of our bodily reactions, we draw away from the signals our bodies are sending. Yet, the heightened sensitivity of pregnancy is a state we should always try to approach. It is to be truly present in our bodies. To explore this, massage therapy or other forms of body-centered work such as yoga, t'ai chi, or physically-oriented psychotherapy can be very helpful.

The type of health care a woman receives during pregnancy will either emphasize or diminish the split between body and self. Traditional health professionals may treat the pregnant woman as if she has a medical condition that only they can understand and treat. The woman is not given a fair chance to develop either the sensitivity to or the trust in what her body can tell her. Luckily, more common these days is the kind of pregnancy care that emphasizes a woman's active involvement. When you are encouraged to take responsibility for making decisions and caring for your body you befriend your body and can begin to take advantage of the wisdom it has to offer.

The sudden awakening of the body in pregnancy comes as a shock to many women. The rapid and intense physiological process pulls our awareness down into our growing bodies. The body comes alive with passion and impulsivity. The stirring of life astounds and amazes the body we may have taken for granted. Hence, the return to the body must proceed with caution. A body that has never been listened to does not trust at first and will not immediately let go of its secrets. It takes patience and kindness to close the gap between body and mind.

There is no particular way in which you should feel in your body in pregnancy. In terms of the transformation to mother, all perceptions are equally informative. It is not "better" to feel revived rather than tired, relaxed rather than tight, motile rather than solid. During the course of the three trimesters, you will have the chance to experience many different conditions. The object is to notice these fluctuations and try to relate them to your personal experience of becoming a mother. We do not expect to have the body of a mother prior to birth, nor should we expect to possess the corresponding psychological skills.

One way to think of pregnancy is as a series of exercises that stretch us internally. These psychological exercises make the self nimble and flexible so that it can form itself around the embryonic self of the child without rupturing. The mother-self snugly and comfortably wraps itself around the baby and holds it tight and secure. The adult's self can contain the child's because the mother has practiced this task daily for nine months prior to birth. The psychological and somatic changes of pregnancy are really the ingenious way in which our psyches are prepared for motherhood.

Fortunately, when you are attuned to your body, you will not only be prepared for the difficult parts of the adjustment to motherhood. You will amply sample the rewards as well. The sensuous body releases intense feelings for the child created out of your own flesh. You are the first person to feel his presence in you body, and you are the first one to know your child. This is an intimacy the father of the child can only catch up with after birth. There are other joys: The hard labor of carrying a child makes you marvel at your own strength. It feeds you confidence in your ability to care for your child once he is born. Being pregnant also brings an incredible sense of awe for life. A human life in all its complexity is formed in your body out of a single egg and sperm, and you are the vessel for this first journey.

To explore further how the pregnant body reflects a woman's changes in self-image, we will use Anna's perceptions.

The Glow of Pregnancy

Mirror! Look! Yes, you reflect the closet darkness most of the time, but today you are filled with me: curves and contours, a full shape, the golden glow of my skin so vibrant I light up your entire surface. Today, I will make such a strong impression on you that you are unable to let go of me. Then, after I leave, you will continue to hold my reflection. My curves and contours will be engraved in you. Perhaps one day when I feel disheartened, you will let me see this beautiful body again; just hold the reflection up to me and let me stand in its radiance.

The glow of pregnancy, that wonderful state in pregnancy when your inner well-being and excitement radiate out through the body, brings an attractive aliveness to your presence. It draws attention to you, eliciting the smiles and compliments of others. The warmth you radiate is contagieous and opens the heart of others.

Examine your glow so that self-consciousness does not cause the feeling to escape and collect as many details about it as you can. Notice what feeds this joy. What gives your heightened sense of aliveness permission to come out? What does it need to thrive? What colors, fragrances, views, tastes, and company surround your aliveness? What body parts generate your feelings of well-being? Collect as much knowledge as you can and store it in an easily accessible place.

Attention

All the people Anna knows have opinions on what they see and advice to give to her. They are absolutely positive that they know the importance of Anna's new body. They know how she feels in it, what she needs to do to it, and what she can expect next from it. They know exactly what is going on now and what will happen to her in the future. More than anything, they know best, simply by looking at her body.

Anna's womb is like a ball tossed between players in a field. Without ever stopping, it flies high up into the air in every possible direction: right, left, up, down, then right and left again. Anna stands by watching. Nobody seems to notice. They have their eyes only on the ball. Anna buries her feet deep into the soil. She will not be pulled into the game. She hates games. She wants to be alone and have her growing womb all to herself. It belongs to her and nobody else.

She loves the attention! Her power to attract is immense. People follow her with their eyes. How could they not? When people look they see something special. Her stout body carries excitement. She glows intensely like the full yellow moon rising after sunset. People raise their heads and look, for a moment forgetting what is on their minds. Anna spreads her white light onto everyone who comes within her reach.

Let them admire her! Let them show their reverence for her! It makes her feel so good, so confident, so proud. She can make an impression by her mere presence and so she will.

There are few life transitions, except possibly marriage, that draw so much attention from others as pregnancy does. Family and friends, as well as strangers, approach you with good-wishes, advice, or speculation about the sex and duedate of the baby. Often it is a welcome topic you love to discuss at length, and you encourage others to share in your excitement. The attention you receive nurtures you. At other times, however, you may wish that your pregnancy were not so apparent and that it would not interfere with matters you consider more important. When you are trying to find your own answers to what is happening to you, you may prefer to do this in solitude and not share the process with the rest of the world. It is important to honor both extremes as valid parts of your experience and to take action to create privacy as well as publicity.

Intrusion

It is eight-thirty in the morning, her hair is a mess, and Anna thinks she forgot to brush her teeth before she left the house. Bus rides are horrible. There are so many people to bother her. "Take it slow, mama!" the bus driver grins when she climbs on. She finds a seat up front. The old lady on her right smiles approvingly at her. Anna gives her a forced smile back. A mother balancing both toddler and grocery bag in her lap asks when she is due. Across from her two businessmen keep glancing at her from top of their newspapers.

Anna is sure the belly button sticks out from her sweater like the cherry on top of a muffin. She tries to button up her raincoat, but the coat is too tight. She crosses her hands over her lap instead. But now it looks as if she is pointing to her oversized waist. If she puts her hands close to her sides, might they give the illusion of slimness? No good. She decides to lean forward and stare through the window instead. Her back hurts, but at least she doesn't have to look at her fellow passengers.

Why should they care anyway? It is none of their business what she hides in her paunch. She wants to be left alone so she can grouch in peace—as she used to, riding the eight-thirty bus without anyone noticing her.

Your distinct body shape is what is most noticeable about you in pregnancy. You cannot shed your protruding stomach when you prefer people not to know about your pregnancy. As you lose your anonymity and become the pregnant woman everyone notices, you also become invisible to others. Your personality seems to fade behind the obvious characteristics of your pregnant body. It is as if others cannot see beyond your pregnancy. What you think and feel are no longer important, unless you want to talk about your baby.

Some women appreciate their new invisibility. They like the opportunity to hide inside and nurture their new mother-self in peace and quiet. For others, their days in cognito feel utterly lonely and confined. They wish more than anything to be acknowledged for who they are, pregnant or not. Again, there is no right or wrong way to feel.

The Powerful Body

Next person who asks to carry her bag she will knock to the ground. How dare they treat her as if she were made of crystal! She is not. She will not fall and shatter into sharp little pieces on the floor. Just look at her body. Her flesh is dense and thick and reinforced by a refined network of blood vessels. She has strong muscles, the kind it takes to carry a child safely. Her weight keeps her standing solidly on the ground. Indeed, her body is more powerful than ever. It will shield and protect both her and her child. It will not let either of them down.

At the same time as a woman may feel more vulnerable than before she became pregnant, she will also feel more robust and powerful. It is as if the extra weight that grounds her in her body makes her feel more emotionally secure as well. To oscillate between the two extreme experiences of the tenuous and the strong is at once thrilling and frightening. Yet the ability to switch back and forth between these two opposites, and even to experience both states at once, facilitates mothering. To care for another being is a most draining task if you do not possess the psychological mechanism that allows you to be receptive and open-minded yet grounded in yourself.

With these examples of how the pregnant body facilitates the psychological adjustment to mother, let us now end this section with some factors that may inhibit the use of body wisdom in the transformation.

THE WAY WE VIEW A MOTHER'S BODY

Although most women are proud of their physical capability to carry and give birth to their child, unease often creeps into the picture in pregnancy as well, similar to what a teenager feels in puberty when her body changes from a girl's to a woman's. All too often the negative feelings dominate the experience. We forget to value the uniqueness of our pregnant bodies. Whether we struggle to keep our bodies as close to the ideal shape as possible, or feminist insights have led us to minimize the importance we place on appearance, the outcome is the same: We do not know how to live peacefully with our pregnant bodies.

Women's unique ability to menstruate and give birth has been viewed with a mixture of awe and fear through the ages. Yet every human being gestates in a woman's womb. The female birth channel is the gateway which brings us into the world, and from the breasts springs the milk we need to grow. Undisputably, the female body makes a unique contribution to the creation of life. The tremendous power inherent in this ability is rarely celebrated. Girls learn early on to regard their female genitals with a sense of shame and disgust. The menstrual cycle is assumed to disabilitate women, making us moody, unstable, and irrational. Commercial interests exploit and reinforce our insecurity by implying that our bodies are enemies we must constantly fight; otherwise we will get fat and wrinkly and emit odors and unsightly bleeding.

Interestingly, research on the female reproductive function sometimes contributes to this negative attitude. In her book *The Psychology of the Female Body*, Jane Ussher[5] explains how much of the work done on female cyclicity focuses only on problems and "syndromes," such as PMS, instead of on what functions can be considered normal and healthy. The disease model of our Western medical system confirms the biological weakness of the female body. It supports the position that women are unable to perform as well as men. Although there is no biological basis for the misconceptions that define women as inferior because of their "bleeding wombs," the belief nevertheless prevails and colors women's perception of their own cyclicity in a negative fashion. Women distrust their bodies, expecting them to cause more problems than pleasure.

Many scholars have described how women on grounds of their biological nature have been restricted from participation in society. Adrienne Rich is one of them:

> The woman's body, with its potential for gestating forth and nourishing new life, has been through the ages a field of contradictions: a space invested with power, and an acute vulnerability; a numinous figure and the incarnation of evil; a hoard of ambivalences, most of which have worked to disqualify women from the collective act of defining culture. This matrix of life has been fundamental to the earliest division of labor, but also, as Bruno Bettelheim has shown, males have everywhere tried to imitate, annex, and magically share in the physical powers of the female.[6]

Although being female no longer disqualifies a person from holding a particular job or political office, the suspicious attitude toward the female *body* prevails. Many women fight the prejudice by minimizing their sexuality. In the professional world, an emotional or physical expression of femininity is not considered an asset if you want to be taken seriously.

In pregnancy a woman's deepest fears about her body are brought out into the open. She can no longer close her eyes to the fact that her physique plays an important role in the new course her life is about to take. She wonders what the implications will be for her: Will her intellectual powers recede? Will fatigue erode her capability? Will she no longer care about anything but her baby? Will other people notice a difference in her? Will they change their opinion of her? Will they treat her differently? Unfortunately, there are some very disturbing realities behind these fears. As a woman's bodily shape gives away her condition to others, people may indeed treat her with less respect. At work she is suddenly defined as a mother, and while her ability and motivation to work may not have changed a bit, her pregnancy may nevertheless affect how employers view her situation and she may be penalized by having fewer opportunities for promotions or salary increases. Such injustices make it hard to welcome a protruding stomach. The expecting mother may begin to resent her unborn child rather than unfair corporate policies.

In view of these depressing social attitudes, let us make pregnancy an occasion when we appreciate our female bodies. Let us remind ourselves that the pregnant body is at a lifetime peak of vitality and strength. Most of the activity takes place in the lower half of the body, the half that is closer to the ground. Whether we are still or in motion, we can draw support from the ground and be focused and efficient in our activities. There is little about the pregnant body that suggests weakness and loss of power. Indeed, our fertile bodies add to our prowess.

THE BODY CONNECTS THE PREGNANT WOMAN TO HER FEMININITY

A woman's body is her most important source of information about the feminine self she may have buried under deep layers of distrust. The body instinctively answers to the feminine self. By tensing up, decreasing or increasing its movements, or making shifts in the breathing pattern, a woman's body speaks up when she tries to override her deeper urges. The bodily reaction informs her of the dangers, errors, or pure dislikes that threaten to interrupt her sense of well-being. Conversely, by pounding with excitement or relaxing and softening, her body will suggest when she is getting close to harmonizing her inner and outer worlds.

The body instinctively understands the female self and translates its character into shapes and movements. The body does not need rational explanations to act out its experiences. It accepts the irrational forces of the psyche and expresses accurately what the mind struggles to conceptualize. A woman may not find that it is fruitful to conceptualize femininity in abstract terms such as "being in touch with your feelings" and "relating to your instincts." Concepts loosely defined soon dissipate into nothingness if they cannot enter the body. But if the woman can experience her femininity in her body, she is offered an alternative to her mental constructs, and she will begin to understand the mysteries of her femininity, first intuitively, then with insights.

The relationship we have with our bodies reveals the relationship we have with our femininity. We may abuse our bodies with drugs and food as well as overactivity or inactivity in an effort to do away with the discomfort we feel in them. We may feel shame over the functions our bodies perform; we may value appearance but have no sense of what our looks convey about our true selves; and we may try to alter the natural size or shape of our physique to fit some external ideal. We may thus forever "stay in our heads" and never look below the neckline to the sensuous world of our feminine bodies.

Our bodies convey our unwholesome attitude toward our feminine nature with astonishing accuracy. We can feel in our bodies whether we berate our femininity (we feel empty, barren, starved, asexual, rigid, and sterile) or whether we are relaxed and comfortable with it (in which case our bodies will feel full, moist, fluid, pulsating, and fleshy).

Marion Woodman describes the woman who has lost touch with the instinctual nature of her body: "She is a soul in search of a body. For the woman, at least, her identity is indistinguishable from her body, and until she learns to look at it as the nourishing source of her feminine identity she will remain out of touch with herself, wandering about in a world alien to her feminine ego.[7] To Woodman, the body is the link to the feminine spirit. Without a positive connection to her body a woman's spirit is caged within the musculature of her body. Every woman must value her femininity by taking responsibility for her body so that it can express the feminine spirit. Our bodies reveal who we are—not what we do, not what we seem to be—but how true we are to our feelings, desires, and values.

When mothering is not anchored in a woman's feminine self, she will lack a firm center from which her interactions with her child can spring forth. Few ideas and impulses will originate within. The woman cannot be spontaneous with her child. She cannot let go and follow the moment. Instead, she will depend on outside influences, such as a particular rolemodel or system of thought, in order to relate confidently to her child. Without such external support, she doubts she will do her child any good. There is little involvement of her true self. In contrast, if the woman learns to mother from her female center, she will participate in mothering with every cell of her being. She will consider her personal feelings, body experiences, intuitions, and every odd idea that passes through her mind important for how she mothers. This gives her flexibility in coping with her baby. She can adjust to what the situation demands. She also appears clear and forthright to her child. There is an "I" meeting "thou" as her child looks into his mother's eyes.

When a woman can accept her body as the manifestation of her feminine soul, the body comes alive. It takes on life with every muscle and bone. Now the woman can openly express the feelings that run through her. Her erect posture speaks of the pride that resides within. Her soft movements demonstrate the sensitivity and care with which she regards herself and others. Her open senses denote her capacity to perceive the subtleties of her inner and outer worlds. She can stand firmly on the ground.

Our bodies also connect us to the feminine on a collective level. Our female bodies carry tradition. They join us to the common themes of all women. Awareness of our bodies transfers to us a nonverbal understanding of the conditions of being born into a female body. Our bodies teach us about the importance of cyclicity in women's lives, of female rhythms and how these cycles can be put to our service. They teach us about female sexuality and its effect on our fortunes. They teach us the power of endurance. They teach us how softness can be as powerful as force. These are truths about womanhood that put us in the service of life.

Our bodies bond us to our own mothers and the sense of trust we as children developed in the safe sphere of our mothers' bodies. The nourishment we received from mother's caresses, the relaxing effect the warmth of her body produced, or the special smells, colors, and rhythms that made her the one and only one are forever kept in the memory of our nerves. The love our mothers showed us with their bodies left an eternal blessing on our organism that sustains us throughout life. When we are in stress, we may without much thought curl up in a certain position or ask to be held in a particular way that comforts us, the same way we were soothed as children.

THE BODY CONNECTS THE PREGNANT WOMAN TO HER CHILD

Your very first meeting with your child takes place within your body right around the day you first begin to feel the fetal movements. From this day you will spin an emotional bond with your child, so that at the time of delivery, you will have established both the readiness and the eagerness to relate to your newborn baby.

The physical experience of the baby in pregnancy is a crucial link to the development of maternal feelings. In a study on the psychological effects of motherhood, Dr. Myra Leifer[8] describes the emerging relationship between mother and child in pregnancy. During the first trimester, most women in her study had trouble visualizing their baby. The fact that the women did not look pregnant promoted their uncertainty regarding the existence of the fetus. The fetus was most commonly viewed as a part of the self rather than a separate entity. Many had a fear of miscarriage, which prompted them to be cautious in investing themselves emotionally in the child. The turning point occurred shortly after the quickening in the second trimester when the mother-to-be could feel that the fetus was alive. The fetal movements became a form of communication between mother and child. Feeling the baby kick and turn, the mother would imagine that the baby was trying to communicate with her. As the affective attachment deepened, the expectant mother began to imbue the fetus with human characteristics and to picture it the way it would be at birth.

The importance of pregnancy as a time of emotional preparation was captured by the women in Dr. Leifer's study after they had given birth: Looking back at their pregnancy, three-fourths reported that they would not want to miss being pregnant; the principal reason was the feeling they had developed for the growing fetus in their bodies. The abstract idea of the baby is consolidated in the body in pregnancy and opens the way for maternal feelings to come through.

After birth, our maternal feelings deepen as we attend to our infants. The way we develop a strong relationship with our babies is rarely a smooth process, and it may take several months for our feelings to reach their full depth. It is, however, through the close and continuous physical contact between mother and child that the emotional intimacy emerges. Physical contact is important for the relationship between father and child as well. Both mother and father intensify their relationship with their child as they hold, touch, and seek eye contact with him. Research indicates that fathers who attend birth and participate in the infant care develop the same strong attachment to their children as mothers, and they subsequently stimulate and nurture them just as well as mothers.[9]

Just as the mother first connects with her child while she is pregnant, so will her child's first experience of mother take place within the security and comfort of her womb. The unborn baby can hear the sound of his mother's voice and heartbeat, his eyes register light, and he can tactilely experience the parameters of the womb he inhabits.

The newborn baby also knows his mother through her body. The words she uses and the thoughts she thinks matter little to him. The infant is closely attuned to the way his mother touches and holds him, the tone of her voice, what she smells like, whether her muscles are tense or relaxed, how she moves, and the way her eyes make contact with his. From these perceptions the infant forms a steady image of mother onto which he can attach his emerging sense of self.

The physical experience of being attended to is the sum and substance of the infant's early awareness of himself. If his experience is pleasurable, he can relax into his mother's body and into his own. He is given a secure foundation upon which to build his own identity. If his mother's body, on the other hand, transmits rejection or if she is invasive or distant with him, the child is prevented from developing a secure connection to his own body. In an effort to protect himself from emotional pain, he seals off these painful emotions by tightening his body. As a result, his self-awareness is cut off from his instinctual body.

Jack Lee Rosenberg, Marjorie Rand, and Diane Asay of the Institute of Body Psychotherapy explain the intimate connection between self and body:

> The sense of Self is a non-verbal experience of wellbeing, identity, and continuity that is felt in the body. If a child's needs aren't satisfied in a loving, caring way, he doesn't develop a strong sense of Self. The potential Self-the undifferentiated mass of energy within the child-remains more or less undifferentiated, fragmented. It lacks the cohesiveness that gives "form" to a person's sense of Self, his identity. This doesn't develop because he doesn't have a pattern of feeling good and comfortable in his body. What he does develop is the character structure of a person who seals off feeling. It is a defensive character structure and the defenses are erected between the Self and the outside world. They are useful in that they allow one to grow without further pain to the Self, but they also maintain the Self in the primitive state it was in when the character structure formed to protect it.[10]

From the child's first day of life, possibly from the day he is conceived, the mother's feelings about herself are transmitted to the child through her body. The way in which she takes care of herself directly affects the formation of her child's sense of self. The child need to experience his mother's well-being in order to develop a healthy sense of self. If his need for love is unsatified, the musculature of his body will seal off the pain he experiences. Over time these muscular patterns become rigid within his body and neither negative nor positive feelings can penetrate his physical armor.

BODY AWARENESS AFTER BIRTH

The boon of body awareness in the mother does not end at birth. Ideally, you will now bring the knowledge you harvested in pregnancy into your role as a mother. During the first confusing weeks with the new baby, your skills at paying attention to your body can help you settle into the mother role: those blue moments come when you cannot figure out what your baby needs, he does not tell you in ways that you can understand, and you get conflicting opinions from your helpers. Panic and despair threaten to overwhelm you. What to do? Ask your body for advice. Your body will give you answers, in its own way. Are your muscles tense and constricted? No wonder the infant refuses to nurse. Does your body yearn to hold the baby although your mother-in-law tells you to leave him crying? Then trust your own instinct and you will begin to know yourself as a mother. Is it because you are a bad mother that you can't stand being with your child one more second, or is it because you are exhausted and need to rest? Do you allow yourself to express the disappointment, distress, and other difficult feelings that belong to new motherhood or does your body silently carry this burden?

You will experience the emotional bond you have with your baby in your body. The sound of your infant's crying cuts through your body like a knife, his signs of hunger stimulate the let-down of milk in your breasts, and his first smile sends warm flashes to your heart. A mother feels her child's feelings as clearly as if they were her own. Yet your body will also remind you that you have adult powers to take care of your child. You can contain the child's feelings in your adult body and take action to help your baby to come to peace.

Your body is the mother of your mental strength and vigor. It not only sustains you but has surplus energy so that you can care for others as well. However, your body does not function well without your love and care. When your own reservoir is empty it is difficult to pay proper attention to others. Finding time to take care of yourself is thus as important as caring for your child. There are many ways to restore the supply of energy to the body. Movement is wonderfully therapeutic, whether it be a relaxing walk, a bicycle ride, a swim in the local pool, or a spontaneous dance to your favorite music. Stretching exercises, meditation, and massage are other ways to nurture both body and mind. Then there is what most new mothers long for more than anything: a good night's sleep.

Chapter 7

A MOTHER'S SEXUALITY

Sexuality is an important part of female identity. It is a source of pleasure and energy that fuels the total personality. Originating in the lower body, our sexuality unites us with our instinctual natures and makes us acutely aware of our innermost likes and dislikes. It is also a force behind our creative activities. We bear our creative projects to fruition, much as we do the child in pregnancy.

Pregnancy and birth are for many women the ultimate manifestation of their sexual and creative powers. It is a time to celebrate the creative nature of the energy that brings men and women together, the deep biological force that motivate us to reproduce. The decision to have a child thus expresses the maturing sexuality, which joins the instinctual drive for pleasure with the drive to reproduce.

Strangely enough, sexuality is rarely associated with motherhood in our culture. On the contrary, mothers are often depicted as asexual beings who are nurturing and loving but hardly interested in sex. If a mother's sexuality is acknowledged, it is thought to belong to her role as a spouse and lover, a role that is kept separate from the mother role. Women's sexual energy is, on the contrary, rarely recognized as a driving force behind mothering.

The abandonment of our sexuality is a significant loss to us as mothers. Sexual feelings can be a steady source of pleasure and well-being that reaches far beyond the bedroom. A woman's sexuality provides strength and energy to the mother role as well. Raising children is a challenging task and it is tragic to lose this form of internal sustenance when it is most needed.

In this chapter, we will explore how a woman's sexuality changes in pregnancy and after birth. We will also see how our attitudes toward sexuality in motherhood affect our relationship to our bodies. Furthermore, we will learn about the power healthy sexuality adds to the mother role.

THE SEXUAL RELATIONSHIP DURING PREGNANCY: A TIME OF CHANGE

Is Anna's body really sexy? How can this disproportionate body, two legs sticking out from under a huge potato-belly, sagging breasts and pudgy buttocks, flabby arms and a swollen face, be sexy? How can she feel so good in her body? Anna laughs to herself. She is the exact opposite of what she has learned to think of as attractive. Not even in her wildest imagination will she pass for one of the slim icons in the fashion magazines.

There is no sense in trying to look different. She cannot change herself. This is who she is right now. And the amazing fact is, she likes herself. She is beautiful! Maybe for the first time since she was a little girl she fully accepts the way she looks. This is not the body she is stuck with until she manages to slim it down into a nicer shape or put on more make-up or buy new clothes. This is who she is, and she is content.

In pregnancy, you are brought into close touch with your sexual body. Genitalia, uterus, and breasts are at the center of events. They dramatically change appearance and function during the course of the nine months of pregnancy. In their central position these body parts receive the full attendance of the feelings you hold toward your entire body. If you are comfortable with your new looks, this can be a time of heightened sensuality, but if you feel awkward, chances are that these feelings will extend to your sexuality as well.

Many women appreciate the beauty of the new fullness of their bodies and the accent it places on their feminine contours. The body feels extra vibrant and alive and affirms the importance of their sexuality for their well-being. They find that they become more attuned to the body and listen more carefully to what feels pleasurable. It feels important to pamper the body a little more, perhaps with relaxing baths, a massage, or fresh flowers to scent the air. The body thrives on the attention. Relaxed and content, it returns a sense of well-being to the self.

For others, the new focus on their sexual organs is not so easy to reconcile. Women are often ashamed of the new visibility of their sexual organs. The lactating breasts look out of proportion and so do the genitalia, and although the reproductive organs are not directly visible to others, they are nevertheless exposed at the many obstetrical examinations. Some women have from an early age been taught to regard their genitals as strange and "unclean." As sites for the menstrual discharge, the uterus and vagina are associated with inconvenience and mess. The cessation of periods in pregnancy may thus be welcomed since it stops the flow of blood, although it was this very function that made conception possible.

Sex can feel very different than it did before in pregnancy and early motherhood. Pain, fatigue, and queasiness will naturally put a damper on your desire. The protruding stomach gets in the way and it progressively becomes more difficult to find comfortable positions during intercourse. The sexual appetite is also affected by the anatomical changes of the body. The genitals may swell from the increased amount of blood and fluids in this area. During intercourse, the vagina may thus feel tighter than before. Touch to your breasts may be perceived as either painful or pleasurable depending on how sensitive and sore they are.

After birth, the vagina is sore from the ruptures and cuts inflicted during delivery, and pain is common when intercourse is first resumed. While a woman is breastfeeding, the low levels of estrogen make the mucous membranes of the vagina dry and brittle. Even if she is sexually aroused, the vagina may thus not become moist and the woman feels sore. It is also normal for the vagina to stretch after a delivery. For some women, the added space gives rise to more intense genital feelings, while others may feel that it is difficult to get the same grip as before.[1]

Some women are concerned about the safety of intercourse in pregnancy. In a normal pregnancy, sexual activities will not hurt the fetus, nor will they cause miscarriage or early labor. The fetus is well protected inside the amniotic sac. Unless the male has a sexually transmittable disease, there is no added risk of infections as long as the amniotic sac is not broken. Only in high-risk pregnancies are there physiological reasons for abstinence.[2]

We have already mentioned how a woman's attitude toward her changing body and self affects her sexuality. Another important factor is her partner's attitude about her growing body. The male sexuality is also affected by pregnancy. Some men are turned on by the changes they see in their partner, while others lose interest in sex during this time.

The conflict and stress that expecting parents experience in their relationship as they adjust to their new roles are often transmitted into their sexual relationship. Unarticulated emotional needs concerning, for example, intimacy and affection can be played out sexually. A man may complain about his wife's lack of interest in sex, when what he really is asking for is his partner's attention, or vice versa.

It is particularly important for a couple to be attentive to their individual differences in pregnancy. Both partners must be sure to articulate their feelings and to be sensitive to their respective needs. One must individually take responsibility for his or her own sexuality, asking for what is needed in terms of closeness and affection, love and sex. Each must also respect the other's right to decline sexual intimacy. It is not advisable to agree to sex in order to please the other partner. This will only build resentment, which prevents the experiences of intimacy that, after all, is more important than sexual activity. The pattern of pursuit and avoidance that follows may prolong indifference to sex.

Ensuring that both partners feel sexually satisfied in pregnancy may take some extra work. A couple must make sure to have time for each other, out of bed, so that they can nurture the feelings that inspire sexual activity. Sexual feelings cannot be forced; they must be enticed. Intercourse cannot be the only measure of how well their sexual life is functioning. The couple can enhance their sensuality instead with lots of body contact, massage, and caressing. There are creative ways to get around the protruding stomach.

If the parents-to-be can be creative about the changes that take place in pregnancy, their sexual relationship will mature and become more integrated into the overall relationship. Both of them may learn to listen better to their bodies. They will become more aware of what they enjoy individually and how to communicate what feels good and what does not to each other. The motivation to experiment and find new ways of pleasure may add new excitement to the sexual relationship, furthered by the fact that for the time being they need not worry about birth control.

THE TRANSFORMATION OF THE SEXUAL SELF IN MOTHERHOOD

Why on earth does Anna feel so exhilaratingly sensuous and sexy now when she is carrying her and Thomas's child? It is almost embarrassing. Now, when she is supposed to become motherly, lust should give in to serenity and virtuousness, for goodness sake, and not erupt like glowing lava from her body.

She is surprised. Why hasn't anyone told her? She knew that some women feel great when they are pregnant, but she assumed the reason was that they were excited about having a child. This is different. These feelings are sexual and not exactly motherly.

Tumultuous hormones? Yes, maybe. Disappears when the child arrives? Possible. But why does she feel so strongly that motherliness and sexuality are connected? Yes, they are. She can feel it from the depths of her body. Her pelvis knows, her womb and her breasts. She must keep this a secret. Few people would understand. It has to be a secret between her and her unborn child.

A woman's first pregnancy marks a rite of passage for her sexual self. From now on, the woman will live in two separate bodies, the motherly and the sexual, the latter kept well hidden from the child. Sadly, it is as if her sexual self is pushed out of body and mind by the growing child in the womb.

The strange division of the body into reproductive and sexual parts confuses women's relationship to their bodies. Breasts, for instance: are they to be regarded as sexual parts of the body, or is their purpose now solely lactation? Is the vulva a gateway to life for the child or a cleavage of pleasure? Unable to fuse the dual functions, new mothers may deny either the sexual or the maternal aspect of their reproductive organs. Some women will not acknowledge that nursing is sexually pleasurable; others find nursing in public embarrassing. Yet others allow the husband's claim to their breasts to have priority over the infant's claim and choose not to nurse for this reason.

Our attitude toward sexuality in motherhood can be studied in the female image of two women, each of whom embodies a side of a woman's sexual self. The two ladies have for ages influenced how the sexuality of women is defined: One woman is wild and voluptuous, the other is innocent and sacred.

A woman's sexuality has an untamed quality to it, represented by the sexy wild woman. This woman is the queen of passion, charged with a mixture of mystery and excitement, bold and explicit in her sexuality. She can be seen caressing her voluptuous body, her full breasts and rounded belly, luring men into sharing her pleasures with hips swaying in intriguing movements. She is the mistress of insatiable lust and eroticism.

In her negative aspect, the wild, sexy woman has another name: whore. This derogatory name reveals our ambivalent attitude toward her: we condemn her for being promiscuous and sinful and say that she is careless and dangerous to everyone. Her powers must thus be carefully circumscribed. She belongs in a pornographic context, where she can be exploited and demeaned, or perhaps, if she is carefully tamed, behind closed bedroom doors. Nowhere else must the sexual self be seen.

As mothers, women prefer not to be associated with someone of such dubious character. How could this wild woman be other than a neglectful mother? This woman is most likely childless, but if she has children they will most likely be seen dangling from her breasts or clinging on to her broad swaying hips while she is out chasing pleasure. Feared and despised, the wild, sexy woman is chased away from the maternal body and out of our consciousness.

Having rejected sexual passion as the raw material for maternal feelings, we are left to make the acquaintance of the other aspect of a woman's sexuality. This aspect appears in the image of an innocent young woman in purest white, her long, soft hair lightly touching her opaque skin. She radiates bliss and serenity, sitting quietly in a stream of silver light that illuminates her benevolent qualities. Her sexuality lies in her sensuality: the tender feelings that are conveyed in her gentle touch and caress.

No one has trouble seeing an infant child in the arms of this lovely woman. Harboring an infinite capacity to love and to soothe, she can be envisioned easily as the ideal mother. Yet most of us will probably deny that this blissful woman is a sexual woman. We associate her with Virgin Mary, who conceived in an act of spiritual purity and not in carnal lust and desire. We regard her chastity as essential to her maternal rectitude. Thus we hardly recognize the madonna's subtle sensuality as sexual energy, especially not in an age where we measure sexuality in orgasmic potency.

No, women of today are not likely to regard the madonnalike woman as a sexual being. We are more likely to recognize her maternal endowments, a role many women have serious doubts about. It is said to be this woman's selfless devotion that turns her children into well-adjusted adults—and we can only commiserate with her heavy burden. Thus, the madonnalike woman's fate is the same as the wild sexy woman's: So long! You are hopelessly prudish and passe.

Both the tender and the rampant aspects of the female sexuality are duly rejected. And so every new mother is left alone with the dilemma of what to do with her maternal, sexual body. Not able to reconcile the two, mothers frequently flee from their bodies. The body is abandoned in favor of the child. Soon they have forgotten to decipher their bodily reactions and pay little attention to what is going on below the neckline.

The loss of a connection to one's body and thus to one's sexuality is a significant loss. When sexual feelings are allowed to surface, they can be a steady source of excitement and well-being that reaches far beyond the bedroom. Raising children is a challenging task and it is tragic to lose this form of internal sustenance when it most is needed.

Is there then no way to entwine sexuality and motherhood, so that we can continue to reap the fruits of being in close touch with our bodily selves, even after giving birth? We could conceivably create an entirely new image of maternal sexuality, but it may be simpler to invite the images of the wild and the innocent sexual woman back into our consciousness and try to retrieve the qualities they represent. With their assistance, body and soul can once again be unified.

First and foremost, we must accept the importance of our female physicality. We must own both the wild, passionate side of our sexuality and the tender, sensuous side and realize that they both belong to us as women. Thus can we adopt the madonna's soft sensuality: how she reaps satisfaction from her relaxed body; how content she is in herself, and how nurturing her gentle, calming presence is. We can also call upon the wild and lustful woman and let her passionate nature infuse energy and excitement into our everyday lives.

In addition to their connectedness with the body, these two females have other qualities worth adopting. We can learn from the madonna's ability to convert her sexuality into the warm and tender feelings that seal her commitment to her children and uphold the emotional connection she has with them. In contrast, the wild woman's characteristic remoteness teaches us the value of detachment. This woman is passionately caring but not necessarily intimate with her children, a position that is called for when it is time to let go and let our children find their own way in life. In addition, acknowledging the wild woman's bold self-expression is important for those of us who believe that a good mother is entitled to only mild feelings.

Why is sexuality so rarely mentioned in the context of mothering that it becomes a source of confusion and even shame? The conflictual attitude must be seen against how women's sexuality historically have been depicted in our culture: "The loss of power associated with woman's sexuality has been a reality across cultures ever since man discovered that he had a role in the procreation of children,"[3] author Maureen Murdoch claims. She argues that women's procreative power, which is so powerful that it can create life, for centuries has been considered a threat to masculine authority. To protect the survival of patriarchal ideals, men would do anything to control women's sexuality, demeaning and prohibiting its expression, even actively destroying ancient goddess figures that glorified female genitalia.

"It is no wonder," Murdoch continues,

> that some women today feel shame about their genitalia and develop sexual "dis-ease," such as condeloma, dysplasia, and herpes. They keep this secret from their family and friends for fear of being considered dirty. They compare the flower of their sexuality to others and find their labia and vagina lacking. Nothing is ever right with their bodies; adolescent girls decry the size of their hips and breasts instead of celebrating their ability to give birth and nurse their young.[4]

In *Of Woman Born* Adrienne Rich also shows how the female body has been viewed, and continues to be viewed, with a mixture of awe and contempt:

> Two ideas flow side by side: one, that the female body is impure, corrupt, the site of discharges, bleedings, dangerous to masculinity, a source of moral and physical contamination, "the devil's gateway." On the other hand, as mother, the woman is beneficent, sacred, pure, asexual, nourishing; and the physical potential for motherhood—that same body with its bleedings and mysteries—is her single destiny and justification in life.

These two ideas have become deeply internalized in women, even in the most independent of us, those who seem to lead the freest lives.[5]

Few contemporary women would agree that their bodies are "their single destiny and justification in life." Yet, our attitude toward our sexuality remains ambivalent. A mother is ideally the altruistic giver who considers the needs of her children before her own. To claim her sexuality would be shocking as it reveals her selfishness: she has strong feelings that do not spring from her love for her children. What if mother has other needs and pleasures than those that are directed at her children? Can she still care for them? Whenever women are viewed as selfless givers, the power of their female sexuality is too threatening to acknowledge.

The original cord,[6] the attachment to our mothers that remains with us as adults and colors our vision of motherhood, is another reason why we have difficulties incorporating sexuality into motherhood. In our childhood memories we usually find little evidence that mother had sexual feelings: mother was about food and comfort and love—she was motherly, not sexy. Naive as it may be, this image of maternity is nevertheless an image we unconsciously conjure when we become mothers ourselves. From this viewpoint, mothers are asexual, because this is how we as children perceived our own mothers.

Generally speaking, we are much more relaxed in our sexuality than our mothers ever could be. However, we continue to receive mixed messages about the desirability of our maternal bodies. It is, for example, interesting to note that the ideal body in our Western society looks so different from that of a pregnant or nursing woman. The voluminous shape of the pregnant body is hopelessly out of fashion. The less expansive and inhabited a body looks, the sexier it is considered.

Having, or desiring, a slim body seems to be a superficial but visible way for us to assert that we have the personal freedom to create and produce that our own mothers lacked. We feel in control when we can shape our bodies to perfection. Unconsciously, we also remain loyal to our mothers, by adhering to an ideal that supposedly will please men. Perhaps the fact that women so readily accept this quixotic ideal reflects not only our desire to appeal to the opposite sex, but also our ambivalent feelings toward our sexuality. We want to look and feel sexy, but will not claim the power that comes with our sexuality. As our mothers were, we are afraid of what would happen if we started to act upon the power our sexual nature provides.

Stepping out of the bath with shining pearls of water on her skin, tiny rills winding down to her feet. The thick terry cloth towel scrubs its pile into the skin. Heat penetrates through every pore. Deep breaths. The rising steam is scented with sweet jasmine and spreads contentment deep into her body.

Anna stands up, leaning slightly backward to gain her balance. This is her new posture. Before she became pregnant, she would slouch forward as if she were trying to cover up her naked chest. Now she thrusts her body forward, breasts and abdomen sticking out, accentuating her femaleness. Her breasts stand boldly out from the trunk, each with one brown eye meeting the gaze of the mirror. Set in motion with her strides they take their own course, swaying and swinging in rhythm.

When she stops moving they too come to a halt, pointing down to the center of her body, as if they were gravitating down in salute to the child they await.

Her fingers leave the soft breasts, following the descending steps of her ribcage. They pause at the base of the round globe that stretches out below. Her hands want to orbit the globe. They glide on the soft surface, up to the landmark of the navel, then slowly down until they reach the dense forest growing in the mouth to her inner body. This moist and warm place is the gateway that separates her inner and outer beings. Through this gateway traveled the seeds that initiated life, and through it will life first enter the outside world.

In the darkness of her inner world, well protected and safe, burns the fire that gives life. It is only natural, she thinks, that this is the place in which her child is created. In here Miriam can snuggle in deep sleep, resting safely in her mother's powerful embrace.

When you know, in your body, the power of your female sexuality, then you will also understand how important it is to bring it into your new role as a mother. This internal fire renders power to warm and spur your entire being. When you keep it alive you have access to an inexhaustible source of energy that is yours to use as needed whenever you nurture, create, love—live.

When you can feel the center of your sexuality in pelvis and breasts, the very parts that nurture the child, you are in direct touch with your instincts. The strong connection will help you to trust your motherly actions. Feeling what you do is right from the depths of your body gives confidence. Your sexual self nourishes the child as well as yourself. The infant drinks of your power, falls asleep in your comfort, and awakens to your strong presence.

What is it like to be the child of a mother with a strong sense of her own sexuality? Obviously, mature sexuality knows appropriate boundaries and does not foster incestuous feelings or acts. It is not expressed in any way that would be harmful for the child. In the context of motherhood, female sexuality is an inner state of mind.

A mother who accepts her sexuality gives a powerful message to her child: Value the body that gives you strength and pleasure. Seeing the pride his mother takes in her own body, the child learns to hold his own body in high esteem. When he is old enough to discover his own sexuality and looks to his mother for her reaction, her acceptance instead of shame will give him a good foundation for his emerging sexuality.

A mother's attitude is important for daughters and sons alike. Girls need to identify with their mother in order to feel comfortable in their own sexuality. Boys need their mother to model the opposite sex, so that they will later know and respect the sexual differences in their adult relationships. Lastly, and what may be most important of all, a mother who acknowledges her own sexuality presents her children with a way to look to themselves for a sense of well-being and confidence.

Sexual energy sizzles and flares, and, like fire, it is not quite predictable. It enthralls us, but it can also scorch our vulnerable soul. We have every reason to treat our sexuality with the same respect and caution with which we treat fire. The ego can be carried away on the rising hot air and become so light, so light. The higher the ego rises the less connected to the inner self we become. All we will care about is to stay up, up, circling carefree on currents of hot air. We no longer listen to life down under.

Sexual energy that works in our service is carefully contained. It is allowed to warm and excite but not to consume. Our body provides a natural container for our sexual energy: it absorbs our excitation and spreads the energy from the genital area throughout the body and out through the limbs. The more open the body is, that is, the less chronic tension it holds, the more energy can flow through it. We can use the energy to love, to act, to be.

"Many men and women mistakenly believe that if they experience their sexual energy, they must do something about it—they must perform, act it out, discharge it. Since having sexual energy is simply a function of being alive, all they need to *do* with it is *experience* it,"[7] say psychotherapists Jack Rosenberg, Marjorie Rand, and Diane Asay.

Sexual energy is not limited to genital sex. Sexual feelings are ever-present in the healthy body as a continuous source of pleasure. Sometimes the feelings are strong and directed toward someone, sometimes they are just a source of contentment within the body. It is the latter aspect that is present in motherhood.

Chapter 8

MOTHER ALONE, PARENT TOGETHER

Parenthood is a joint venture of man and woman. Although this book is a study of the female transformation to mother, we must not forget that the experience is just as vital to a man's sense of self as it is to a woman's. In this chapter we will therefore make an effort to understand the male transformation to father. We will also examine the issues impending fatherhood awakens in the pregnant woman.

The old man, having raised four children, took pride in the fact that he had never changed a diaper in his life. I cannot remember that he ever rolled wet snow into a snowman or lifted his stiff neck to watch white animal clouds glide over the summer sky. He could not. He had said good-bye to childhood forever the day his drunk mother got after him with the rolled-up newspaper once more. He swore he would never treat his kids as he had been treated, and he never did. He was a good father, he really believed he was, and Thomas kept quiet about the ways in which he had failed him.

It's not that the old man did not teach Thomas about fatherhood. He taught responsibility, values, and commitment. It's just that Thomas does not want the same things he fought so hard for. Now, in the short time that is left until he will become a father himself, this is truer than ever. He does not want to be an outsider as his father was. He wants to know his children. He wants to see them grow with his own eyes. He wants to hold and play and cook for them long before it's time to take them to the ball park. He has a vision, just as his father had. And Thomas is as lonely as his father was in making his dream come true.

One of the most disheartening facts that children who are brought into this world face is the disturbingly low odds that they will be loved and cared for by their father. More than 40 percent of all children will spend their childhood in single-parent families. In 1990, every fourth child was living with mother only, compared with 5 percent in 1960.[1] Too many children will grow up with the painful truth that their father abandoned them. Many more will claim they never knew their father. *The absent father* is a concept as commonly discussed in the context of family life as it is prevalent in our culture.

A father is absent when he does not live with or visit his children. He is also absent when he works eighty-hour weeks or when he is at home but not interacting with his children. His absence leaves a pit of loss and longing in his children. Without his father, a son loses his most important role model for masculine development. He loses the person who can best teach him how to handle the impulsiveness and aggressiveness that come with his masculine energy. Nor is he offered the psychological guidance he needs to make the leap from mom's lap to the outside world. This leap translates into important steps toward independence such as inner direction and intentionality, autonomous action, and personal values.

The daughter of an absent father is also deeply betrayed by her father's absence. She is deprived of a parent who can encourage her competence and inspire her self-confidence. As an authority figure, a father optimally gives his daughter an experience of consistency and fairness. He helps her understand limits and have realistic expectations. As a member of the opposite sex, he affirms her sexuality and shows his appreciation of their gender differences. He can help set her free of society's narrow definitions of womanhood and encourage her to explore nontraditional areas for women. He also teaches her about men's trustworthiness and commitment to relationships, and this affects how she will handle her own intimate relationships later in life.

Statistics provide us with the most convincing arguments for why fathers should be involved with their children. Paternally deprived individuals are overrepresented among the population with psychological problems. More than 70 percent of all juveniles in state reform institutions come from fatherless homes. Teenagers with absent fathers are twice as likely to drop out of high school.[2]

There is currently a surge of commitment to change the traditional distant/absent father role. Men want to be involved in fathering their children, women want them to, and together they are willing to work toward shared parenting. Pregnancy is the first stage in the making of a parent. It is at this early point that we must identify the obstacles to the male transformation to father. In the following section, we will examine some of the early struggles of fatherhood.

THE PREGNANT FATHER

If someone asked Thomas what it was like to expect a child, he would probably make a joke about the perils of living with a pregnant woman. If the inquirer then said "No, seriously, what is it like?" Thomas, embarrassed, would have to reveal his uncertainty. Yes, for sure, he is going to be a father, but not until later, after his child is born. He does not know how to expect a child.

So he pretends. He takes his wife to the gynecologist, he asks the doctor the right questions, and he keeps quiet about how the sight of blood makes him sick. He keeps it together. He lets Anna be pregnant.

But the uncertainty does not go away. What is he supposed to do with his feelings? He does not even know whether they are normal or if he is the only father-to-be who is confused about what it is he is supposed to be doing in pregnancy.

Once a man has planted his seed in the depths of a woman's body his direct participation in his child's growth must wait until after birth. Throughout the following nine months his contact with his child is mediated through his pregnant wife. If he seeks perceptible reassurance of his child's existence, he is reduced to putting his hand to his partner's stomach to feel the miniature limbs press against her abdomen or to watch the shadows of the child's movements travel over the stretched skin. His prepartum interactions with his child are triadic at best and sometimes involve a fourth, technological medium, such as the stethoscope or ultrasound scanner.

The father-to-be lacks the biological affirmation that makes parenthood imminent and real in a woman. A man's experience of becoming a father must instead rely on abstract reasoning and imagination. The unborn child lives in his father's mind only. The abstract nature of their connection to each other makes the man's transformation seem far more uncertain than his partner's. Unless he consciously initiates the process, pregnancy will be a psychological moratorium for him, a waiting period without much activity aside from the occasional visit to the clinic or the Lamaze classes.

Pregnant woman. Pregnant wife.
So beautiful. So full of life.
Sitting in the rocking chair,
sitting in maternity.
Rocking our child to sleep
the gentle, rhythmic, peaceful way
the way she found in pregnancy.

Pregnant woman. Pregnant wife.
Do you even know I'm here?
Sitting in the rocking chair,
sitting in maternity.
You are turned toward yourself,
the way you found in pregnancy.
Pregnant woman. Pregnant wife.
I thought I knew you. Now I don't.

Men often acknowledge that they feel unimportant and excluded during pregnancy.[3] In comparison to the attention paid to the pregnant woman, men's thoughts and feelings are often trivialized. Everyone asks how the mother-to-be is doing, but few remember to ask the father-to-be the same question. The expectant father's role is often defined as that of support for his wife. To add to the feeling of exclusion, men commonly feel they are being ignored by their pregnant partner. In the midst of her pregnant self-preoccupation, the wife seems to have lost interest in her husband in favor of the child.

A man's feelings of exclusion can unwittingly slip into indifference. In an essay on fatherhood, Jack R. Heinowitz[4] cautions that without any real appreciation for his own growth process in pregnancy, the father-to-be may take a back seat at this time. He may focus exclusively on the needs of his pregnant wife or he may immerse himself in activities away from home. Thus he perpetuates the role of outsider. Such patterns may easily continue after birth. In what he calls the "glass-ceiling" at home, Dr. Shapiro describes the negative circle that ensues when fathers play the role of the second-class parent:

> As a man I am not expected to set policy or to make decisions. I carry out orders. In such an inequitable situation it is natural for me to avoid extra work and to revisit the old army rule, "Never volunteer." A psychological cycle is set in place. I play the role of the "lazy husband" to my wife's role of "nagging wife." Neither of these roles is attractive, satisfying, or desirable.[5]

The man's role in pregnancy may be more elusive than the woman's but it is nonetheless equally important. The marital relationship undergoes many changes during this time and needs special attention from both partners if it is to endure the stresses of the transformation. The risks are well documented. Of all divorces 50 percent occur during the child's first year and 50 percent of these children lose contact with their father.

Family life begins in pregnancy. During this time the emotional context in which the child will grow up takes shape. A man can join his wife to create a warm and welcoming atmosphere for their child starting in pregnancy. With his presence or absence, support or debility, the father-to-be indirectly influences his child in utero. The feelings that flow between the two parents are transmitted to the child via the mother.

THE MALE TRANSFORMATION TO FATHER

Thomas thinks he knows what it takes to become a father. It takes a man of conviction, who does not lose track of his vision even when his manhood is at stake.

There lives in him a man who is determined to test his commitment. He asks tough questions. "What about your career?" he asks. "You are just about to get a promotion. Are you going to let that opportunity slip out of your hands? Your boss will get the wrong idea if you tell him you want to take time off to be with your new baby." He tries to tell him he is irresponsible. "You cannot afford to mess up your career right now," he argues. "Soon you will have a whole family to feed."

When Thomas envisions himself playing with his child, the voice inside, agitated, no longer tries to appeal to reason. He hears him whisper, "Boys don't play with dolls and men don't play with babies."

The fact that most men will make their debut as all-out parents as soon as their child is born has dramatically altered the importance of pregnancy as a time of preparation for men as well as women. Until recently, it was difficult to find any accounts of expectant fatherhood, except the token description of the conspicuous couvade symptoms found in some men.[6] The few records one would find of early fatherhood skipped pregnancy and started at the birth of the child. For example, Martin Greenberg began his 1985 account of fatherhood in *The Birth of a Father* with a touching description of the exhilaration he felt as he attended the birth of his first son. He cited this deeply affective moment as the moment that sealed his commitment to be closely involved with his son.

In the scheme of events, birth is probably the most powerful in the making of a father. This is the father's true meeting with his child, a moment he will likely never forget. Yet, although the delirium of birth makes one forget what preceded the event, the process of becoming a father starts at a much earlier point. Becoming a father is a gradual sequence that simmers in the male mind all through the nine months of pregnancy.

Expectant fathers, like expectant mothers, experience a broad range of feelings related to the prospect of having a child. Stepping into the unknown territory of fatherhood may elicit a man's fears and insecurities about his abilities. The man may wonder what kind of father he will become and how his child will perceive him as a father. He may also feel ambivalent about his new commitment. Fatherhood may well bring happiness, pride, and a new sense of meaning to life, but it also means a loss of freedom and egocentrism.

During pregnancy expectant fathers develop a feeling of protectiveness that Jerrold Lee Shapiro claims is almost universal.[7] The sense of responsibility for his family can take many expressions in a man: from anxious concern about his wife's eating habits and general health in pregnancy, to a rearrangement of his professional goals, to a realization of home-buying plans. Undoubtedly, the protective and providing functions are remnants of the days of rigid role divisions when mothers worked at home and fathers went to work outside. We can even go as far back as the days when men were hunters and women nurtured land and children. Despite the restructuring of our social roles, men apparently continue to feel responsible for the financial security of the family. In pregnancy, the pressure to perform may thus be felt with accentuated intensity.

Only recently have we come to regard parenting as a task that is best shared by men and women. Most men grew up with the idea that mothers were the natural caretakers. Mothers, and mothers only, possessed the magical maternal instinct and tender feelings that small children needed. Fathers in turn were supposed to show their youngsters the way of the world. The latter is still true for fathers, but to a lesser extent. Working mothers are also role models for their children.

That fathers are not as well equipped to take care of their infants as their wives is a long-lived myth in our society. Up until now, so much emphasis in the advice given to new parents has been on the mother-infant relationship. The expectant parents learn about the emotional bonding that takes place when the baby is breast-fed and held close to *the mother*. It is the father's job to facilitate the motherchild symbiosis, and, by implication, he can best do so by taking on the protective role. Little wonder if men feel redundant and awkward with their infants; at least in the past they were never encouraged to take care of them on their own.

With the exception of breast-feeding, there is little evidence to support the notion that the biological predisposition of women makes them more competent parents than men. Research shows that men who care for their newborn babies read and interpret their child's behavior and respond to their needs as competently as mothers.[8] Social mores, not biological imperatives, determine which parent is more likely to take care of the infant. Yet, if new parents continue to believe that fathers are less important to their infants than mothers, they have little reason to change the peripheral role of the new father.

Although a father can make up for lost time later in his child's life, something valuable is lost when he does not get to know his child in infancy. In the tender moment of the one-on-one meeting between parent and child, love springs forth. Martin Greenberg calls the new father's infatuation with his infant *engrossment*:

> Engrossment refers to a father's sense of absorption, preoccupation and interest in his baby. He feels gripped and held by this feeling. He has an intense desire to look at the baby, to touch and hold him. It is as if he is hooked, drawn to his newborn child by some involuntary force over which he has no control. He doesn't will it to happen, it just does.[9]

Presence and availability are the magic elements that open the new parent to feelings of love and affection. The day-to-day acts of caring transform the insecure and uninvolved adult into a confident and interested parent. Competence is a direct result of one's presence. Warm feelings do not grow and mature into love when we are not there.

THE MODERN FATHER

Miriam, I want you to know me as the guy who smells kind of musky like a pine forest after it rains and who has a voice that murmurs like thunder down in his belly and then rolls out of his mouth and, magically, reaches your tiny ear as a tender whisper. I want you to know me as the guy who plants kisses on your cheek, and while they tickle—it is called a beard—you know they are just for you.

I want you to know me as the guy who makes the room light when it is dark and you are afraid, the guy who also understands that tumble dryers can be very scary. I want to be the one who shows you buses and escalators and merry-go-rounds. I want to be the person you want to be with when Mom is out.

What I have just said is just the beginning. Later, I want to be the guy who teaches you about life.

If we could remove all premeditated notions of what make a man a man, what characteristics would remain that makes fathering different from mothering? In the sixties and seventies, many argued that intrinsic male/female dispositions simply did not exist. If we could only rid ourselves of the habit of labeling our behavior as masculine or feminine, man and woman would emerge as two androgynes. In terms of parenting, the only sexual difference would be the anatomical difference that grants women the exclusive right to pregnancy and nursing. Psychologically, a man is equipped to be as receptive to his children's needs as any woman.

The father who emerged from the sexual revolution of the sixties could put away his John Wayne imitation. He was free to show his children that men too can be soft and gentle. In Jungian terms, he had discovered the womanly feelings of his "anima," his feminine soul. The idea of neutralizing the genders did not remain popular for long. Currently most seem to argue that the differences in the way men and women are cannot be eliminated no matter how gender-neutral we become in our attitude. We are better off accepting the uniqueness of each respective sex.

It is not so difficult to understand why the unisex ideals went out of fashion. The particularities of man and woman allure and inspire us humans. We make love, create, and rejoice in the energetic field that exists between the two polarities. In Sam Keen's words, the question of gender is penultimately a problem, but ultimately a mystery:

> So what's the difference between a man and a woman? I can't say, but that doesn't mean that I can't recognize the difference. A genuine mystery is protected by silence that remains after analysis and explanation. We approach the mystery of our being by respectful listening, by recollecting our experience, by cherishing paradox and, above all, by loving what we cannot reduce to understanding.[10]

Jungian analyst Anthony Stevens[11] argues that although men and women can function in each other's roles, that is not what they constitutionally are best equipped for. The role differentiation rests on an archetypal foundation that predisposes men and women to act differently and this shows up in the parenting roles. The mother dominates the realm of feelings, instincts, and the unconscious: that is, the aspect of life (and our personalities) that does not evolve over time. The father, on the other hand, represents consciousness as it moves and changes with the outer world. A father acts as a centrifugal force that orients his children toward the world, whereas the mother is a centripetal force drawing them toward the home and the family.

Although it is difficult to determine what is an effect of traditional role patterns and what might be considered a true gender difference, it is nevertheless interesting to note how a couple typically adjust to each other in teaching their children the different movements of life. The possibility of teaching one's children about opposites and contradictions in a clear way is much greater when two people act out one position each. Parents complement each other and give their children examples of diverse modalities of being. However, in the spirit of psychological wholeness, each parent must also possess the characteristics of the other in himself or herself.

In reaction to the earlier "feminization" of men, Robert Bly, a respected spokesman for the current men's movement, laments:

> There's something wonderful about this development—I mean the practice of men welcoming their own "feminine" consciousness and nurturing it—this is impor-tant—and yet I have the sense that there is something wrong. The male in the past twenty years has become more thoughtful, more gentle. But by this process he has not become more free. He's a nice boy who pleases not only his mother but also the woman he is living with.[12]

Robert Bly argues that the modern man lacks the resolve to say what he wants and to stick by it in his relationships. As a father, this kind of man is a powerless and dispirited role model for his children, and although he may be more involved with his children than previous generations of fathers, he is overshadowed by his "strong and liberated" wife.

Sam Keen, another powerful voice in the discussion of modern manhood, has a strong reaction to labeling the tender qualities of a man feminine:

> I can locate nothing that feels "feminine" about holding my daughter in my arms. . . . As nearly as I can tell, I, being a man, have nothing feminine about me. For me, feeling proud of being a man involves practicing the virtues of repentance, compassion, patience, carefulness, etc. My virility is inseparable from opening out, receiving, embracing.[13]

What men currently seem to be saying is that they are not satisfied to mimic the way their partners mother. As fathers, they want to have their own dignity. They want to express kindness, love, loyalty, and so forth, in the family in ways that are true to them. The Modern Father, then, has stepped down from the superior position on the father/king throne and up from the inferior father/servant position on the floor and now wants to be seen as a father with his own parenting style.

Jerrold Lee Shapiro, who interviewed over eight hundred fathers in surveys in the late eighties, came up with a list of twelve core factors of modern fathering.[14] First among the core traits is the protective and providing function, which still seems to be essential to the male image of fatherhood. Other traits include the father's ability to be encouraging and supportive, courageous, trustworthy, and loving with his children. He also lists the fatherly tasks of administering discipline, demonstrating teamwork, and honoring his own and others' personal limits.

One aspect that both men and women seem to be ardently searching for in themselves at present is their "wild, undomesticated natures." Compare the following quotes by two immensely popular authors, Robert Bly and Clarissa Pincola Estes, who have successfully captured the psychological longings of the modern man and woman, respectively:

> When a contemporary man looks into his psyche, he may, if conditions are right, find under the water of his soul, lying in an area no one has visited for a long time, an ancient hairy man. . . . What I am suggesting, then, is that every modern male has, lying at the bottom of his psyche, a large, primitive being covered with hair down to his feet. Making contact with this Wild Man is the step the Eighties male or the Nineties male has yet to take.[15]

> No matter by which culture a woman is influenced, she understands the words *wild* and *woman*, intuitively. When women hear those words, an old, old memory is stirred and brought back to life. The memory is of our absolute, undeniable, and irrevocable kinship with the wild feminine, a relationship which may have become ghostly from neglect, buried by overdomestication, outlawed by the surrounding culture, or no longer understood anymore. We may have forgotten her names, we may not answer when she

calls ours, but in our bones we know her, we yearn toward her; we know she belongs to us and we to her.[16]

Both the Modern Mother and the Modern Father, as they emerge out of the men's and women's movements, seem to share some basic concerns. They are determined to *be present* in their family life; they are willing to go spelunking into the darkest caves of their selves in order to become better parents; and they wish to parent in a soulful, earthy manner.

With these reflections on the mother-father mystique, we will leave the male transformation to father and again turn our attention to the female experience of pregnancy.

FATHERS AND THE TRANSFORMATION TO MOTHER

In an essay included in an anthology on the father-child relationship, feminist author Sarah Maitland writes:

[Father] is alive and well and rampaging inside me. He never goes away, although sometimes he is silent; he is never ill, never weakened, never leaves me alone. He lurks about under other names—God, Husband, Companion—and all those relationships are made possible (which is nice) and impossibly difficult and conflicting because of the father who is in and under and through them all. In my late teens I fled my father's house; it has taken me a long time to realize that I carried with me the Father from whom I could not escape by escaping childhood, from whom I wrest my loves, my voice, my feminism, and my freedom. It is this Father that I have hated loving and loved hating. It is this Father I want to kill, and dare not.[17]

The father Sarah Maitland so vividly describes is not her biological father but her *internalized image of her father* as he appeared to her when she was a child. Within her every woman carries her own unique father image, a clone of the personal and the archetypal father. The internalized father remains a powerful influence on a woman throughout her life. Just as the adult daughter continues to have an invisible and often unconscious umbilical cord that links her internally to her mother, so she has powerful emotional ties to her father as well. He is extremely important to her view of herself as a woman. Only in relation to his masculinity does her womanhood make sense.

The inner father is particularly opinionated during the transformation to mother. In the ultrafeminine state of pregnancy, the father imprints in the female psyche greatly affect how the woman feels about herself during this time. Any judgments she may have internalized about being a woman in general and a mother in particular will emerge.

The role of the internal father is to *follow* the woman on her journey into motherhood. The inner mother is her guide, the inner father her companion. He is at once the illuminating "other" that gives contour to the feminine "self" as she emerges in motherhood and a powerful source of self-love who either undermines or supports the transformation.

Ideally, the father gives his blessing of his daughter's pregnancy when she still is a little girl and not when her pregnancy is fait accompli. The father who appreciates his daughter's budding femininity and conveys his acceptance congruently in his feelings and actions gives his daughter a gift for life. *The woman she one day will be* has his permission to be herself whether it be in her relationships, work, or motherhood. He gives her permission to value that which sets the two of them apart: her capacity to bear children. With his sanctions, the adult daughter will feel entitled to express her femininity in the mother role.

Fathers transmit to their daughters their personal relationship to women and also the cultural view of motherhood. The extent to which the father managed to challenge the cultural stereotypes of women will in turn determine how multifaceted and rich his daughter's initial perception of herself as a mother will be. If a woman has inherited a narrow, two-dimensional facsimile from which to mother, she will have to do much work to ensure that her relationship to herself and to her partner gains further depth and meaning in pregnancy.

The inner father affects how a woman relates to her physical self in pregnancy. If she in general feels strong and healthy, she probably is fortunate to have internalized the message from her father that she can trust that her female body is capable and powerful enough to carry a child. The woman who is plagued by sickness may be fighting an internal father who sees pregnancy as an opportunity to vent his aggression against the female body. The inner father also affects whether the woman feels sexual or asexual in her pregnant body. Many fathers transmit the notion that motherhood and sexuality are incompatible in a woman and that sexual feelings in pregnancy are shameful.

The masculine strength a woman has available in pregnancy determines how independent she can be in making practical decisions. There must be a part of her that can separate from the passive, gestating woman whose entire focus is on the child. The father-inspired part of her protects her vulnerable self. It sees to her needs and realizes them in the outer world. This is the protective and assertive function of the father archetype which the woman carries within.

In his negative aspect, the inner father may interfere with a woman's decisions regarding career and family life. Whenever there is a conflict between her personal desires and the ideals she grew up with, the woman can expect that a pinch or two of emotional discomfort will spice up the decision-making process. If a woman has modeled her professional life after her father, she may find it extremely difficult to see her pregnancy as anything other than a distraction from more important work. Alternatively, if she has internalized the belief that a woman's place is at home with her children, it may be difficult for her to hold on to a career after she gives birth.

A woman's ties to her internal father contribute to the general tone of her pregnancy and also equip her with some important coping strategies to help her get through the experience. The masculine mode complements the ultrafeminine gestation. Being passive and yielding may come very naturally to a woman in pregnancy, but she must also have the inner strength to assert herself with firmness and authority. As she falls into the self-absorbed haze of pregnancy, she needs a countersource to pull her into reality again. If the inner father is either too weak or too disrespectful to stand tall in the presence of this feminine energy, his light may not shine through. The woman is helplessly drawn deeper and deeper into the dark side of the feminine with confusion and emotional exhaustion as the results.

Pregnant women carry the self-denigration they inherited from their father in different ways. One woman may be so overwhelmed by the negative feelings her ultrafeminine mood elicits that she at any cost must deny the impact pregnancy has on her. As far as it is possible she acts as if she is not pregnant. She turns her interest to projects outside herself and will not miss a beat of her usual pace. Another woman may not be able to ward off the pregnant mood, but since she devalues her feminine experience, she is engulfed by anxiety. She feels at the mercy of her feelings, hoping for someone to piece her together again. The physical disturbances of pregnancy may stay with her longer than normal as they amplify her helplessness.

A third woman may have such difficulties accepting the leadership of her feminine willpower that she protects herself by "getting pregnant" instead of consciously making the choice to be pregnant. Unconsciously, she may well wish to express her feminine self in relationship to a child, but her negative sense of self forbids her to have such feelings. Tragically, the demonic internal father wins the battle and her pregnancy is fraught with resentment.

Let us take the subject of the internal father's influence in pregnancy into further depth by examining two different stances women typically take in pregnancy. Both are a result of the early relationships these women had with their father. The first stance is illustrated by the woman who feels most comfortable with herself when she can emphasize women's similarities to men, the other by the woman who is most comfortable expressing the differences between the sexes. Different as they may seem in the life-style and values they honor, we shall soon see how similar their underlying attitude to their feminine selves in reality is.

THE FATHER'S DAUGHTER

The Father's Daughter is a character we know from the previous chapter on femininity. She is the "modern woman" who on an egolevel identifies with the masculine. She has adopted from the male world the professional ambition and leadership qualities that one rarely would see in women at the time she was a girl.

The Father's Daughter will only like herself when she is tight, bright, and light. Her psychological tightness allows her to hold her own in the man's world. Her brightness is a measure of her well-developed intellectual capacities. The lightness in body and spirit signifies that she has succesfully liberated herself from the maternal roots she dislikes. Yet, tightness in a negative sense is a sign of the hardening of the ego, of armoring, bitterness and pent-up feelings. Likewise, brightness brings little satisfaction if it is not connected to the inner self, and mental lightness leaves a woman ungrounded and thus susceptible to the ever-shifting winds of public values and opinions.

The pregnant woman softens and rounds out psychologically and physically. She is far from the ideal tight, bright, and light woman. This is an experience that the

Father's Daughter has tried to escape all her adult life. In pregnancy she stands face to face with the immense power of her irrational, emotional self, and she is terrified. This is her Achilles heel, the weakness she fears will puncture her powerful ego. She does not know how useful the unpredictable nature of her unconscious can be, for she has never been shown how to have a fruitful relationship to this part of herself. Her father feared and devalued the mysterious feminine, and she learned to do the same. He did not know how to relate to the feminine, nor does she.

The foremost transformative task of the Father's Daughter must be to become comfortable with her pregnant personality. She must realize that women who use their femininity to mother have a softer and more malleable strength than the masculine forcefulness she is accustomed to, but it is not less effective.

Linda Leonard calls the woman who has formed a psychological armor against her femininity an "Amazon Woman." She describes the healing process in which the woman comes to appreciate her femininity in the following passage:

> The Amazonic woman has already developed a lot of strength and power in her life and this is very valuable. The issue is rather to allow that strength to come out natural from the center of her personality rather than be forced out from an ego adaption. What is needed is to bring that strength to the area of which she is afraid. It is neither a weakness to be in the irrational realm nor to use it as a source of knowledge. To the contrary, it is a weakness to be unable to face this aspect of life. If the Amazon woman can learn to value her vulnerability and the uncontrollable aspects of existence, she may find a new source of strength. The creative process offers many examples of the necessity to go down into the unconscious and remain there in weakness, perhaps in depression, boredom, or anxiety, in order to bring up the "new being," the creative attitude which can change one's life.[18]

The transformation to mother may have the unexpected benefit of putting the Father's Daughter in touch with her feminine warmth and wisdom.

DADDY'S GIRL

The father-daughter relationship of the woman who is a Daddy's Girl is distinguished by a sweet and innocent flavor. There lingers in the adult daughter a feeling of preciousness that stems from her father's love and devotion to her. However, her self-esteem is conditional. The girl-woman must act in a certain way that suits her internal father in order to like herself. In pregnancy she may act fragile, compliant, or always happy, just as she did as a little girl. She acts "as if," because she does not know how to be herself.

For a Daddy's Girl, becoming a mother involves a struggle toward autonomy and individuation that rearranges the ties with her internal father. Psychically, her pregnancy bears special significance: Daddy's Girl is now a woman bearing another man's child. She can no longer be little, a girl, or daddy's. Two responses to the separation are possible: Either the woman experiences her pregnancy as if she has fallen from her father's grace and feels guilty for having broken the unspoken agreement that her father and she would always be there for each other, or she grasps pregnancy as a chance to liberate herself from her past. The transformation to mother will therefore bear many resemblances to teenage rebellion.

The other possible course Daddy's Girl can take in response to her pregnancy is to remain loyal to the unconscious agreement she has with her father. Since her self-esteem is dependent on her acting in ways that please her internal father, she becomes the kind of mother that her father would approve of. The precious girl becomes the revered Madonna. The new mother continues to feel special as long as she mothers in ways that fit the idolized image of motherhood. Should she fall short, shame and self-hatred would surge forth.

The woman who shares some of the characteristics of the Daddy's Girl must sacrifice her attachment to her feelings of specialness, since these feelings come at a price that is much too high: If she continues to act as a loyal daughter, she will not find her own power as a woman and as a mother. Instead, she must become aware of the shadow side of her father's love for her: first, the conditions stipulated to his love, and the egocentricity with which he rules over their relationship; then, his insensitivity to her feminine self and his tendency to impose male values that in effect demean her as a woman.

The loss of the original father relationship is a loss of innocence that is painful but necessary if the woman will be able really to value herself as a mother. If the woman can let go, her pregnancy can be a true spiritual pregnancy; a time to discover her true potential at a slow but yielding pace. Her relationship with her child will then be mediated by a *benevolent innocence*. Her emerging mother-self can meet the child in a spontaneous sharing of their uniqueness.

THE FATHERLESS DAUGHTER

Absent fathers also leave their daughters with well-defined parameters for their transformation to mothers. The father who abandoned his family left his daughter with the legacy that men do not find women worthwhile when they mother. The career father who was never at home conveyed the message that the world of work is much more exciting than staying home with a child. The deceased father leaves his daughter with a deep longing for a father figure who can help her define her role as a mother. In all three instances, the women will have unrealistic expectations of motherhood.

The woman who has been physically, sexually, or emotionally abused by her father is also a fatherless daughter. A man who violates his daughter's integrity is not fathering her, he is destroying her selfhood. The abusive father teaches his daughter that as a woman she is worthless and deserves to be poorly treated. During times when her femininity is augmented, as it is in pregnancy, the woman is prone to self-hate and negativity.

FORMING A NEW FATHER RELATIONSHIP

The original relationship to our father, which we continue to reenact in the present, must be transformed in pregnancy. A woman cannot claim her own power and independence as long as she remains loyal to this early relationship. When her internal father holds the authority, her choices as a mother are limited. Either she will obey and become the mother her father desires or she will oppose him and become everything he detests. Either way, she will mother in relation to his authority.

Every woman needs a healthy inner father to enhance her feelings of self-worth in motherhood, for "a healthy inner father is like a reservoir that makes us feel full, generous, and calm."[19] Thus the pregnant woman must attempt to heal the wounded father in her heart.

The healing process involves a series of steps. First, she must become aware of the emotional wounds of her personal father. She must recognize the destructive attitudes that were transmitted to her through him. Second, she must understand how this mind-set affects her feelings about becoming a mother in the present. This includes untangling her fantasies about what a man expects from a woman who is a mother, and also what she as a mother hopes to get from a man.

Father hunger[20] drives women's expectations of parenthood as well as men's. Most women have grand expectations of their husbands as fathers. The husband should provide everything the woman did not get as a child: a loving, involved, interested, attentive father to their child. He should be there for her as well: the attentive, involved, interested, and loving partner she needs to mother well. Simultaneously, she may expect him to provide financially for her and the child: to be a rock of support and a succesful businessman all at once. Other women prefer their husband to stay away so that they can enjoy the power that comes with being the family matriarch.

The pregnant woman must consider how her vision of fatherhood serves her psychological transformation to mother: What kind of mother will she be if she, for example, believes fathers are (1) omnipotent, (2) worthless, (3) critical, (4) submissive? What kind of mother will she be if she continues the pattern of her parents' marital relationship? With insights into her tendencies to hold on to the past, the woman is better able to make positive choices for her own parenting experience.

She must also come to see the value of her personal father, because his healthy aspects are hers as well as his wounds. Behind all the hurt is most often a father's genuine love for his daughter. The mother-to-be who is able to forgive her father for his shortcomings will also soften the self-critical attitude that cannot accept her own limitations as a mother.

MOTHER ALONE, PARENT TOGETHER

"Hello, is anybody there?"
"Sorry, of course I am here. What did you ask me again?"

"This happens all the time. You are here allright, but you just walk around with this vacant look on your face and I have to repeat everything I say at least once. Sometimes I wonder if I have done something wrong."

"Just because I am quiet doesn't mean that I am sulking. I feel fine. I'm just not in the mood for any lengthy conversations right now."

"Well, I had to ask. It feels sort of awkward between us these days. I just don't know how to be around you."

"Just be yourself."

"Then I have to be honest and say that I feel that you really do not want me around, like the baby is yours only and I don't have anything to do with it. And our child is not even born yet!"

"That's not true. You know that I want us both to have this child. But I often wonder if you want to be around. Like you are so committed to our child?"

"Because I think about our child and I want us to have some extra money when the baby is here. I call that commitment, don't you?"

"To me it looks like you are running away."

"I can't believe this conversation. What is it? Some competition for who will be the more devoted parent?"

As we have seen in this chapter, fatherhood is a subject both men and women dwell upon in pregnancy. For a man, pregnancy is the start of his own transformation, with the triple focus on the past, present, and future convening in the process of becoming a father. For a woman, pregnancy revives her psychological ties to her own father, which in turn shape her expectations of her husband. For both of them, impending parenthood brings a whole new dimension to their relationship.

In many ways it would be easier for a couple to accept the traditional pattern of parenthood in which men are the distant providers and women the nurturers. But such strict role divisions promise to be disappointing. These traditional roles do not satisfy the desire of most parents to give their children a different kind of parenting experience than they had. Shared parenting is also a financial necessity for most people dependent on a dual income. Thus, the parents-to-be become pioneers in the largely unexplored territory called shared parenting. And the differences in opinion, territorial fights, compromise, and negotiations begin.

Children are our second chance to get close to what we did not get for ourselves as children. That is why we are prepared to fight so vehemently with our partners to stake out the rules and responsibilities. We simply wish to match our own parenting style with the missing pieces in our psyches, and this includes our partner's parenting style as well.

"I'm sorry. I didn't mean to push you away. I want you involved. This is our baby, and we are both going to be there for Miriam, just as we decided in the beginning."

"I am sorry, too. I should have talked to you sooner. I lost it there for a while."

"It's frightening, isn't it, how easy it is to fall into the roles we both want to avoid

as parents: I am having a cozy old time with the baby while you feel left out."

"You are pregnant; I am not. It's hard to avoid at this point. We just have to be careful so we don't get stuck here."

"It's scary how comfortable it feels to me, to continue in the tradition in which we were raised."

"But we both want it to be different and we must not lose track of that."

"Maybe there are some things we can do to get you more involved in the pregnancy."

There is no shortcut to shared parenting. It helps to have a thorough appreciation for the difficulties the parenting revolution contains. With empathy and compassion, a couple can pave the way for an open-hearted discussion of what they must do to realize their vision.

Parenthood requires a renewal of the marriage vows. In sickness and in health, the couple promise to support each other as parents. The marriage is the place where both can find strength and enthusiasm for their parenting.

Chapter 9

THE WISDOM OF THE WOMB

"Thomas, the water broke."
"What?"
"Here, on the floor. I felt a warm gush run down my legs and when I looked down there was a mirror of water on the floor."
"What does it mean?"
"I am in labor."
"What do we do now?"
"Thomas, you have read all the books as well as I have! You know what to do, don't you?"
"Yes. Yes, I do. Are you in pain?"
"No, I don't feel anything. Let's go back to bed for a while."
"Will you wake me up?"
"Yes."

As pregnancy draws to an end, you gain perspective on the psychological transformation that has preoccupied you for so many months. You are now at a point where you can look back and see how the first elusive signals of change have matured into an explicit declaration of intent: At nine months pregnant, you are unmistakably with child.

The preparation that takes place in pregnancy enables you to open up to that which is yet new and unknown. You have let go of your old self. You are in the final stage of a long period of internal shedding what is irrelevant to your new mother-self. At this point, but rarely sooner, you are ready to take responsibility for your desire to mother *deliberately*. Although you long ago reached a point of no return, this deliberateness of intent seals your preparedness. You can affirm your transformation:

I want to be a mother. I accept that as a result of this wish I will change. I will change in a way that will reflect my own way of mothering my child.

In stating to yourself your *desire* to be a mother, you accept motherhood as a conscious decision that you are willing to take responsibility for. Making yourself accountable for your desire is a way to get truly excited about birth. You permit yourself to focus all your mental and emotional energy on this one event. You are full of child. You also declare that you are willing to *change* to accommodate your child. Inexperienced as you will be, you give yourself permission to be a scholar in the art of child rearing, recognizing that you must take every chance you come across to learn how to mother your child. Lastly, you *search* for a way to mother that is right for you. You vow to make sure that as a mother there will be more of you and not less.

In order to find your mother-self, you must temporarily shut down your antennae to the outside world. Then you are free to go deep inside and ask yourself, Given who I am, what I think, feel, and what is most important to me, what kind of mother do I aspire to be?

Why search within for an image of good mothering? The reason, unfortunate but real, is that *mother* as she is represented in our collective consciousness so often is a sorry character. Where will pregnant women find a "role mother" in society, who inspires rather than exhausts their ambitions to mother well, who reassures rather than daunts their confidence, and who challenges them to get into the heart of the matter rather than to polish their exterior? Not in media: the TV and film mother is too unrealistically portrayed to be of value. Not in feminist literature: mothers are all too often used as a warning example of what can happen to a woman if she gives in to convention. Not in history books: perhaps they will find some positive aspects of the mother in ancient mythology, but the vicimized mother dominates the scene.

Women are in dire need of a positive model of mothering that will match the free-spirited, competent woman of the nineties. This new model is yet to be created. It becomes the responsibility of every new mother to envision motherhood with fresh eyes. The woman must turn inward to the heart of her feminine self, where, whether she is aware of this yet or not, there awaits a wealth of good mother wit.

This final chapter is dedicated to the wisdom of the womb, which simply but crucially is a source of internal guidance that every woman has title to. Out of this inborn wisdom arises a mother image that will challenge any dismissive attitude toward mothering. First, however, we shall briefly explain why it does no good to look to society for the emergence of the New Mother.

At quarter past nine, as the pale November sun crawls over the rooftop, Anna finishes her second cup of tea and the two pieces of toast Thomas insisted that she eat. Next to her on the kitchen table stands her new canvas bag. The three zippers on the bag are neatly closed. The tag she attached to the handle displays her name, address, and date of birth. Anna does not know it yet, but she will many times unzip the tote bag only to zip it up again before Thomas finally grabs the bag in one hand and sticks his other under Anna's arm and leads her to the waiting car. She will empty out the contents of the bag, double-check that she has everything on her list, repack the suckers and the music tapes and the address book, carefully making sure the most important items lie on top and her slippers and robe are at the bottom. But for now she can think of nothing to distract herself with. She has already showered, put on her most comfortable clothes, and, while listening to the morning news on the

radio, watered all her plants. She tried the TV, the phone, and the newspaper, but
she is too restless. All she can do is to wait for the next contraction to besiege her.

Thomas checks on her every once in a while to see whether there is anything he
can do for her. He pretends to be reading the newspaper, but Anna knows that he is
watching her closely. Every time she leans against the wall or the table top he is
there, anxiously timing her contraction.

"So this is it," she thinks. She is only hours away from becoming a mother. She
is preparing to step into the limelight that surrounds women who devote themselves
to the young.

Our contemporary world is confusingly ambivalent toward motherhood. On the one
hand, a mother is praised and honored for her priceless contribution to society's
renewal. On the other hand, no other role seems quite so unimportant. The expecting
woman may find herself on a pendulum between one extreme, in which maternity is
the ultimate state of bliss, a rosy existence where the mother is a smiling woman
holding her angel baby, all lace and teddy bears and cute accessories, and the opposite
extreme, in which she sees herself as a hollowed-eyed mother drowning in the throes
of a screaming infant, messy diapers, and sour milk. Both of these images borrow their
simplicity and unfairness from our collective stylization of motherhood.

How seriously do women take society's representation of motherhood? Not very,
one would expect, since these images are not directed at one personally and are often
so blatantly exaggerated we can but laugh at them. Yet, in a culture where the nuclear
family is the norm and few parents-to-be live close enough to other families with
children to be let in on the mysteries of parenthood, who else is there to tell us about
having children? Lacking exposure to real life parenting, many of us rely on society's
representation of motherhood as our guide. It may seem that these accounts would give
a benign introduction to the mother role, perhaps even be the best way to get an
objective picture of the pros and cons of parenting, if it were not for the sad fact that
the majority of them present a derogatory view of mothers.

Our society is quick to blame mothers for its many problems, whether it be the
high suicide rate, criminality or drug abuse. *Mother blaming* is a socially acceptable
way to vent our frustrations over life's miseries. As Dr. Jane Price says:

> Society feels free to spell out what it thinks is "good mothering" and to judge and
> condemn women who fall short of those criteria without feeling any obligation to pro-
> vide practical support, encouragement or reward for the job. This split between the
> power to influence and the acceptance of responsibility for the consequences causes
> much bitterness in women, who feel quite literally left "holding the baby" on behalf of
> everyone else.[1]

What are the cardinal mistakes a mother can make that will make her fit for blame?
The negative attributes that describe the flaws of the horrible mother roughly fall into
two categories: Mothers are either ruthlessly powerful or feebly incompetent.
Whichever category a woman falls into is not important, both will label her
detrimental to her offspring. Let us briefly study the two opposites as they can be seen

in the Omnipotent Mother and the Martyr Mom, each woman with her distinct set of unattractive characteristics.

The Omnipotent Mother is feared for her unrestrained power over her flock. If she chooses to abuse her power, and you can be sure she will, she can easily damage her children's well-being. When bad things happen to them, it is always of her evil making. She manipulates, cajoles, and instigates to get her way with her children, who have nothing to do but obey her commands.

Another of the regrettable characteristics of the Omnipotent Mother is her utter selfishness, also referred to as her narcissistic and hysterical tendencies. This witchlike mother unashamedly uses her children for her personal gratification. She achieves her personal goals without any concern for their needs. Like helpless puppets, the children move to the pulls of her strings, unable to assert their own will. Selfishness not only describes the mother who is overinvolved in her children's life, but also the mother who does not spend enough time with them. To pursue one's own interests, to choose work over homemaking, and to hand over the caretaking to a husband or baby-sitter is socially condemned on the grounds that the mother's decision will have severe repercussions for her children. Paradoxically, society is also often suspicious of a mother who is very devoted to her children. Surely she must have hidden motives for her involvement? Is she really doing what is best for her children or is she merely fulfilling her own needs at her children's expense? The bad Omnipotent Mother seems to lurk behind every happy mother.

The Martyr Mom lacks the arrogance of the Omnipotent Mother, but her behavior nevertheless causes her offspring great dismay. The Martyr is the great sacrificer. She demands nothing for herself, but lives to fulfill the needs of others. She is the woman who is stupid enough to believe she can live up to the celebrated mother ideal. Making no attempt to break away from her fruitless endeavor, she suffers quietly and ceaselessly. It is mainly the Martyr Mom's daughters who are the victims of her poor mothering. With such a weak role model in their lives, they are prevented from becoming confident and self-loving women themselves. Slowly but surely they are engulfed by their mother's martyrdom.

The Omnipotent Mother and the Martyr—both deliver a depressing prospect of motherhood. As a mother, you will be scorned and shunned; you will be isolated and lonely; nobody will take you seriously; and you will destroy your children. What, grim fate, is in store for you? These stereotypes certainly do nothing to build confidence in the mother-to-be. How can she trust that she will be able to mother and to do it well, when there are so many stories that advise her of the hazards? Who will support her, who will applaud her efforts, who will believe in her? Why should she bother to become a mother at all?

In times like these, a woman has to distance herself willfully from the mainstream or she will be infected with its cynicism. The new mother cannot afford to be undermined. She is in search of the power and self-confidence she needs to nurture her child and nothing must stand in her way. It is *that* important. She needs to go where life is valued for what it is.

We should not fool ourselves into believing that we can and should cut all ties to society, hoping that as long as we are connected to our inner selves, we will be strong, happy, nurturing mothers. We are social beings who must cope with the external reality. We need a society that validates our deepest emotions and truest thoughts. We need acknowledgment for who we are and what we are doing—especially when we mother.

Jane Swigart speaks of the *holding environment,* a term borrowed from D. W. Winnicott, with which she means to point out that the nurture and support a child needs extend beyond the mother's arms to the entire ambiance of the world that surrounds them:

> If a mother is not given a protective, supportive "holding environment" for herself as she tries to provide for her infant, her relationship to the young new life can become painful and traumatic. What is traumatic for the mother is traumatic for the infant, baby, and toddler. I am convinced that a supportive "holding environment" for care-givers requires a compassionate understanding of the mother's deepest feelings, as well as knowledge of the external realities with which she must cope.[2]

We must accept that we are social creatures and that we need society's support as mothers, but we cannot expect society to present us with a novel interpretation of the mother role. *The new mother* must be born outside convention and the only ones who can do her justice are people like you and me, who are willing to appear a little bit crazy in order to give motherhood a new face. We are the women who can ignore the raised eyebrows and the sullen murmurs we will meet, or imagine we will meet, whenever we do something differently. We are brave and determined and prepared to work hard to embody our vision. We listen inward and when the time is right we share our discoveries with the world.

Having justified our lack of interest in the external world during the transformation to mother, we are now ready to go where life is nourished as it is. We are ready to turn our attention to the imagined center of our feminine self—the womb.

There are powers inside stronger than I have ever known, trembling and quivering to force me to admit that in their presence I am never fully in command. With the rise and fall of each new encounter I bow, in awe and apprehension.

I am drawn into the epicenter, where no one else will ever be able to accompany me. I leave Thomas behind. Only his hand remains in my awareness. I can feel the dry palm of his hand stroking my sweating back with little circular movements. It is only me now and my wilfull body breathing and contracting as we reach the peak together.

Just when I know I cannot take it anymore I am suddenly released from the grip, like a wildcat, who, tired of playing with its prey, will sometimes release rather than kill it. Soothing waves of mercy roll in and I am allotted time to imagine how the crown of the baby's soft head now rests against the brim of my pelvis.

Slowly the room returns. I can see the armchair with the two citrus-colored pillows that really do not go well with the earthtone of the forest-green upholstery. Under the coffee table, the stack of magazines has tipped over to form a glossy puddle on the floor. I can even see a gray coat of dust on the poster frame above the

chair. How I welcome this familiar room. The objects in here reassure me of their
continual allegiance. No matter what I will experience in the following hours, when
I return they will still be here.

The womb is a rich metaphor for a woman's ability to bring forth new life. By
studying how the womb acts toward the fetus in its care, we can learn vital lessons that
help us once it is our turn to be in charge of the caring.

Unquestionably, seeking the counsel of one's belly is not an ordinary way of
approaching the art of mothering. We are not used to regarding the womb as anything
other than what it is anatomically: an organ of the female reproductive system. Few of
us think of our lower body as a plausible source of information about ourselves. Not
to worry if consulting the womb seems a preposterous undertaking. Having a belly
protruding an elbow length out from the body makes it virtually impossible to miss its
significance. We can see with our own eyes that mothering revolves around our lower
bodies. Our minds follow suit. In late pregnancy, most women are preoccupied with
what is going on down under.

The Swedish word for womb is *livmoder:* "mother of life." The womb mothers new
life until it is ready to be born. To become a mother is to be initiated into the mysteries
of the life-bearing womb. By respecting her innate wisdom, the new mother learns
what life needs to thrive. As the womb does in pregnancy, she will now nurture and
protect her firstborn.

The womb is our origin. It is the vessel from which we all were born. The womb
fulfills the conditions we need to grow from a fertilized egg to a fully developed human
being. The uterus is a hollow, muscular, and urn-shaped organ that lies well protected
in the cavity of the pelvic bones. This is the ideal environment for the creation of
human life. As mothers, we can strive to be womblike. We can assure ourselves a
space clear of poor advice and false pretense in which we are free to grow strong and
healthy, and we can erect strong psychic walls that, like the uterine wall, will protect
our woundable selves from harm. Furthermore, we can let rich soul blood nourish us
and wash us clean of debris and foreign matter. In this way we take care of the
newborn mother-self.

The womb carries the archetype of The Great Mother,[3] a collective image that
every human being knows intuitively. The Great Mother is a power beyond us, greater
than any human mother. She forms and transforms human life. She is the origin of
human consciousness. When we draw wisdom from the womb, we draw wisdom from
a source deep down under, a source that listens to the spirit of Mother Nature. "The
person with the most power is the one who can most deeply allow life to flow through
her to others," says Carol Wallas LaChance.[4] The image of the Great Mother teaches
us to honor our connection to all life on earth.

The nameless woman whose laughter shadows the contraction like the murmur
of thunder rolling off a hilltop—this is her glorious day, during which she undisguised
will show off all her talents. "I have no fear," she shouts, "Nothing can stop me. I will
accomplish what I am destined to do."

When in a moment of doubt I wonder how I will get through to the end as I am still only in the opening stage of delivery, the madwoman is there at my side. "Breathe with me," she says, "and I will take you through." In breath we meet. We are no longer strangers to each other. We share a common goal, and that goal is birth. Each deep inhale I take refreshes me and in each exhale I find relief. The madwoman shrugs.

The womb is the seat of our instinctive selves. As we have seen, the rational part of a woman's psyche is submitted to the irrational throughout pregnancy. Spurred by hormonal and physical changes, impulses and emotions get a chance to govern our behavior. These are characteristics of the soul untamed: the animalistic, unsocialized self that hides beneath our normally level-headed exterior. The madwoman within—why is she allowed to dominate in pregnancy? Why does she appear at a time when the mother-to-be needs clarity and sound insight into the mothering role? What, if anything, does this wild woman have to do with mothering? She apparently bears little resemblance to the calm and serene woman most of us envision as the ideal mother.

The womb-woman keeps us connected to our instinctual nature. To act instinctually is to act from the center of one's being, from the inner self that knows how to make a woman thrive and therefore is in the best position to determine in what ways a woman must rearrange her life in order to come into her mother-self. Will you be a better mother if you become an earth mother or a woman with diapers in her briefcase, a homebody or an entrepreneur, a playground keeper or a day care expert? There is no general formula that can answer these questions. Our choices as mothers have multiplied in number during the last decades, but if we are to be enriched and not savaged by them, we must know what is right for *us* personally. To borrow ideas in our surroundings is wise, but the final saying must come from the wise woman of the womb.

The irrational, womblike woman deglorifies motherhood. She helps the mother-to-be understand the double nature of all mothers: how the nurturing and caring mother also can be raging, suffocating, resentful. She exposes the unsuspecting mother to the negative side of mothering. In her refusal to idealize motherhood, the madwoman inside inspires the mother to be realistic about her abilities. She reminds the new mother to be aware that her dark shadow not fall on her vulnerable child. Real mothers are human, often wonderfully loving like the Great Mother in her nurturing and protective function, but sometimes they are not. Acknowledging one's humanness is not an excuse for a mother to be reckless but a reminder to be aware of one's destructive potential.

The madwoman who emerges from the waters of a woman's unconscious will continue to bother her with uninvited impulsiveness and emotional outbursts until she finally is taken seriously. She is vehement in her beliefs and steadfast in her determination to provoke internal changes. Full of warmth and passion, the womblike woman infuses the new mother with the strength she needs to stay off the beaten track. Yes, it is possible, she says, to bring happiness and satisfaction into a role so often depicted as suppressing and depressing.

The insanity of new motherhood is not just a by-product of the psychological adjustment to a new and demanding role. This state of mind is also what makes the new mother so closely in tune with her infant. The wild mother in the psyche understands children. She knows what is good and harmful for a young soul. She cunningly nurtures and protects the free spirit of the child, because she herself cannot live without this freedom.

As we now understand, the irrational is an important force in the transformation to mother. The new mother has no choice but to treat her insanity with love and humor and to recognize what it contributes to her new understanding of herself.

My child, very quietly you tumbled through the cosmos of my womb and embedded yourself in the soft and welcoming lining. It happened so calmly that I did not become aware of the promise you made at that time, that as long as you would continue to grow in me, the woman you had chosen to bear you, you would touch my life in ways that only gradually would be revealed to me.

Now, a short year later, we are ready to meet each other. I give you my blessing on your journey into the world of light and life. This is our first and most important separation. Only by letting go of each other can we finally meet. You leave behind a lasting impression in me. My womb will bleed out of loss. Slackened and vacant it will begin to heal itself, while I prepare to greet you.

I want you to know, my child, that even before we meet you are my most treasured gift. I will try my very best to ensure that you will always know the beauty you are.

When pregnancy draws to an end, the womb releases the life it has nurtured to maturity. At the same time, the mother-self is born. The wisdom of the womb will now belong to the mother. She is responsible for bringing its lifegiving powers into the world so that the child can continue to thrive. The wisdom of the womb extends out into the world through the mother. The mother nurtures her child's sense of self until the child is ready to cope on his or her own.

A woman's ability to recreate the conditions of the womb in relation to her child is illustrated in the following passage by Kathie Carlson:

> In a predominantly positive relationship, the mother creates an emotional and psychological "container" for the child which, like the literal uterus during gestation, has both boundaries and flexibility, growing with the daughter until she is ready to move out of the maternal container into a larger world. Rules, limits, familiar rituals, and endearments define the parameter of this container, while empathic companioning and spontaneity enable it to be flexible and adapted to the child's shifting needs.[5]

While we understand that the child needs a long time both inside and outside the womb to reach maturity, we are rarely so patient with ourselves. We cannot wait for the baby to be born so that we can try out what we have learned about infant care; we lose our internal focus to the quandary of preparing for labor; we may even attempt to skip these preparations, scheduling the personal transformation to take place after birth so that we can go on as usual for yet some time. In our impatience, we forget that the inner transformation to mother is a creative process that needs time and seclusion. It cannot be hurried. It cannot be forced. Only when we allow ourselves to search for the right conditions will dramatic changes take place.

The womb is far removed from the reflective mind. Its wisdom is not highbrow and abstract but rooted and concrete. What is not experienced in the tissue simply does not exist to the womb. It is only concerned with what is growing inside and has no interest in the world outside. The wisdom of the womb is therefore not enlightening as learning new facts or making new associations is to the mind. Receiving its knowledge will not likely cause a woman to exclaim, "Oh, I see, so this is how it works!" The womb nourishes in the dark and its wisdom remains obscure. The woman's response to the womb's teachings is more of a nod of recognition than an exclamation. "Yes, this is the way it is," she may say. Something feels right to her, although it may not be immediately apparent why this is so.

The womb does not ask, What good is the child, whom I am creating, to me? The womb holds no hostility to life. It treasures life for simply being what it is. When we make its wisdom ours, we are able to accept our most original expressions of motherhood without abhorence. Thus we release our creativity. We grow as mothers when we respond with creative solutions to the constantly changing conditions of parenting.

One way to recreate the unconditional acceptance of the womb in our daily lives is to meditate. To meditate is to practice the art of being. Linda Leonard says:

> Meditation is a practice in which one attends to being in the moment. It transforms [one's] tendency to lose the genuine gift of life in fantasies of the past or future. When one meditates one dwells with the presence of what is. Thus, one can respond to the gift of that moment of life. Meditation is a practice of letting go. One sits, attending to the breath, and allows what appears to be and also allows it to go. [The] tendency to cling to people, places, or things, to try to control and possess, is surrendered. Through this meditative attention to being, clarity arises. One can finally see in the mirror of one's being.[6]

When we master the womb's way of being in the present moment, we also open ourselves to be with the child. We see into the mirror of the child's being as well as our own.

There are other ways to clear oneself from unnecessary clutter than to meditate. A *plain and simple* living cultivates the art of being.[7] The daily care of an infant—feeding, diapering, napping—fosters one's appreciation for the moment. Simplicity is not boring when it is seen as significant.

How does the womb create? Science can show us in detail how the female body carries life from fertilization to birth. With the help of fiber optics we can see the process with photography that "quite literally illuminates the mystery of pregnancy without in any way diminishing its splendor."[8] Yet, science cannot explain all. How does one come to life? There is still much that has never been documented. The womb instructs us that we must surrender to the life force, whether we understand the process or not. In labor, we surrender to the womb. The womb contracts, relaxes, contracts until it has completed its mission and the child is born. We participate in the nativity, but we do not necessarily penetrate the process with our minds. The mysterious forces of nature prevail.

The Hebrew word for compassion/mercy, *rachamim*, comes from the root word of womb: *rechem*. Therefore we can say that a person who is compassionate is a womblike person. The passionate energy that flows from the womb fuels a mother's love for her child. She generously offers the child that which is vibrant in her; she shares her loveliness with her infant.

Erich Fromm identified four basic elements of love in his classic study *The Art of Loving*.[9] These are care, responsibility, respect, and knowledge. "Love is the active concern for the life and the growth of that which we love," he said. Care and concern in turn imply responsibility: a loving person responds to the needs, expressed or unexpressed, of another. Responsibility could easily deteriorate into domination if it were not for the third component in love: respect. To respect another means to be concerned that this person should unfold as he or she is. Finally, Fromm said, to respect, be concerned about, and take full responsibility for a person would not be possible without knowing him: that is to see the person in his own terms.

The compassionate womb carries the propensity for the expression of these four elements of love. It cares for, it respects, it knows about new life. The maternal impulse to love one's child is rooted in these basic instincts of the womb. A woman is wise to treasure them.

Quietly Thomas drapes the coat over Anna's shoulders. As he sticks his one hand under Anna's arm and picks up the red canvas bag with the other, he asks Anna:
   "Are you ready?"
   "Yes," she answers. "I am ready."

NOTES

CHAPTER 1

1. Thomas Gordon, *P.E.T.: Parent Effectiveness Training* (New York: Wyden, 1970).
2. Jane Price, *Motherhood: What It Does to Your Mind* (London: Pandora Press, 1988).
3. Jane Swigart, *The Myth of the Bad Mother* (New York: Doubleday, 1991).
4. Carol Dix, *The New Mother Syndrome* (New York: Doubleday, 1985).
5. Gunilla Eldh, "Spädbarnets skrik avslöjar mamman" (article on Dr. Ann Frodi), Dagens Nyheter (Sweden), December 15, 1991, part 2, p. 14.

CHAPTER 2

1. Sally James, "Too Precious Parenting," *Mothering*, Summer 1990, pp. 25-29.
2. Marion Woodman, *Addiction to Perfection* (Toronto: Inner City Books, 1982), p. 52.
3. Angela Barron McBride, *The Growth and Development of Mothers* (New York: Harper & Row, 1973), p. 16.
4. Read more about values in collision in Joyce Block, *Motherhood as Metamorphosis* (New York: Dutton, 1990), chapter 5.
5. Estimated fertility rate 1990-95. Projection by the United Nations Population Fund (UNFPA). *The Universal Almanac 1994*, ed. John W. Wright (Kansas City, Miss.: Andrews & McMeel, 1994), p. 335.
6. Elisabeth Badingter challenges the existence of maternal instinct in her controversial book *Mother Love: Myth and Reality* (New York: Macmillan, 1981). She argues that mother love is socially conditioned and varies with the mores of the times. The idea that women should be mothers first and foremost emerged in the last third of the eighteenth century with Rousseau's romantic view of childhood as man's natural and savage state, she claims.
7. Alice Miller, *For Your Own Good* (New York: Farrar Straus Giroux, 1980), p. 257.
8. Colette Dowling, *Perfect Women* (New York: Pocket Books, 1988), p. 5.
9. Ibid., p. 60.

10. The role mother is a woman with experience who can model to the newcomer what mothering is about. Unlike the ideal mother, she will reveal her humanity, her weaknesses and mistakes, as well as her strengths.

11. For a pragmatic discussion of the psychological theories on our emotional needs, see Thomas Paris & Eileen Paris, *I'll Never Do to My Kids What My Parents Did to Me!* (Los Angeles: Lowell Books, 1992).

12. Ibid., p. 92.

13. Jack Lee Rosenberg & Marjorie Rand, *Body, Self, and Soul: Sustaining Integration* (Atlanta: Humanics Limited, 1985), p. 20.

CHAPTER 3

1. Joyce Block, *Motherhood as Metamorphosis* (New York: Dutton, 1990), p. 190.

2. See, e.g., the writings of the French feminists Simone de Beauvoir and Elizabeth Badingter. Simone de Beauvoir, *The Second Sex* (New York: Vantage Books, 1989), Elizabeth Badingter, *Mother Love: Myth and Reality* (New York: Macmillan, 1981).

3. As the femininist theorists Chodorow, Gilligan, and Dinnerstein have shown, the development of the self is different in men and women. For example, boys must separate from their mothers and identify with their fathers, thus making independence and separation their primary developmental task, while women develop in the context of sameness. Nancy Chodorow, *The Reproduction of Mothering* (Berkeley: University of California Press, 1978). Dorothy Dinnerstein, *The Mermaid and the Minotaur* (New York: Harper & Row, 1986). Carol Gilligan, *In a Different Voice* (Cambridge, Mass.: Harvard University Press, 1982).

4. Block, *Motherhood as Metamorphosis*, p. 182.

5. Sally B. Olds, Marcia L. London, & Patricia A. Ladewig, *Obstetric Nursing* (Menlo Park, Calif.: Addison-Wesley, 1980).

6. Evelyn R. Duvall, *Family Development* (Philadelphia: J. B. Lippincott Co, 1971).

7. Beppie Harrison, *The Shock of Motherhood* (New York: Scribner, 1986).

8. Vangie Bergum, *Woman to Mother: A Transformation* (Granby, Mass.: Bergin & Garvey, 1989).

9. Andrea Boroff Eagan, *The Newborn Mother: Stages of Her Growth* (Boston: Little, Brown, 1985).

10. These authors include Marion Woodman, Jean Shinoda Bolen, Polly Young-Eisendrath, and Linda Leonard. *To be a Woman—the Birth of the Conscious Feminine*, ed. Connie Zweig (Los Angeles: Jeremy P. Tarcher, 1990), is an anthology that includes essays of these and other authors interested in the feminine. The themes of the book center around the emergence of a new feminine consciousness.

11. As defined by Sukie Colegrave, a Jungian psychotherapist, in *To be a Woman—the Birth of the Conscious Feminine*, pp. 19-26.

12. Ibid., p. 214.

13. Maureen Murdoch, *The Heroine's Journey* (Boston: Shambhala, 1990), p. 7.

14. Robert A. Johnson, *Femininity Lost and Regained* (New York: Harper & Row, 1990), p. 6.

15. Myra Leifer, *Psychological Effects of Motherhood* (New York: Praeger Publishers, 1980), p. 167.

16. Connie Zweig, *To Be a Woman—the Birth of the Conscious Feminine*, p. 9.

17. Marion Woodman, *Addiction to Perfection* (Toronto: Inner City Books, 1982), p. 98.

18. Jean Shinoda Bolen, *Goddesses in Everywoman* (New York: Harper & Row, 1985).

19. Clarissa Pinkola Estes, *Women Who Run with the Wolves* (New York: Ballantine, 1992).

20. See, e.g., Merline Stone, *When God Was a Woman* (San Diego: Harcourt Brace Jovanovich, 1978).

21. The devaluation of the feminine has been suggested as a contributing reason to psychological problems common to women, such as eating disorders and substance abuse. See, e.g., Kim Chernin, *The Hungry Self* (New York: Harper & Row, 1986).

CHAPTER 4

1. Marie-Louise von Franz & James Hillman, Lectures on Jung's Typology (Dallas: Spring Publications, 1971), p. 138.

2. Nancy Friday, *My Mother, My Self: The Daughter's Search for Identity* (New York: Dell, 1987), p. 53.

3. Kathie Carson, *In Her Image: The Unhealed Daughter's Search for Her Mother* (Boston: Shambhala, 1989), p. 7.

4. Evelyn Bassoff, *Mothering Ourselves: Help and Healing for Adult Daughters* (New York: Dutton, 1991), p. 85. Dr. Bassoff offers encouragment for women whose conflictual motherdaughter relationship impairs their adult functioning. She says: "In order to heal, women who as children were unmothered or under-mothered must learn ways to soothe themselves and to fill up the 'holes' within that have resulted from early deprivations" (p. 121). Dr. Bassoff advises these women to find the affirmation, protection, and nurturance that will compensate for their early losses in healthy relationships in the present. She also suggests that we connect with the healing forces of nature, and she points out how our creative endowments can help us make sense of the void within.

5. Carl J. Jung, *The Archetypes in the Collective Unconscious: Collected Works of C. J. Jung*, Vol. 9, Part 1, Bollingen Series (Princeton, N.J.: Princeton University Press, 1959), p. 189.

CHAPTER 5

1. Lucia Capacchione, as quoted in Jeremiah Abrams, *Reclaiming the Inner Child* (Los Angeles: Jeremy P. Tarcher, 1990), p. 210.

2. Sheila Kitzinger, *Women as Mothers* (New York: Vintage Books, 1980), p. 81.

3. Ibid.

4. Ibid., p. 9.

CHAPTER 6

1. Marion Woodman, *Addiction to Perfection* (Toronto: Inner City Books, 1982), p. 79.

2. Alexander Lowen, *The Betrayal of the Body* (New York: Macmillan, 1967), p. 235.

3. Ibid., p. 236.

4. Compare to the witch Anna meets in Chapter 2, *The Perfect Mother*. The woman fears her maternal body because she identifies her growing body with the dark side of the mother archetype: the side that seeks destruction and disintegration.

5. Jane M Ussher, *The Psychology of the Female Body* (London & New York: Routledge, 1984).

6. Adrienne Rich, *Of Woman Born* (New York: W. W. Norton & Company, 1986), p. 102.

7. Marion Woodman, *Addiction to Perfection*, p. 98.

8. Myra Leifer, *The Psychological Effects of Motherhood: A Study of First Pregnancy* (New York: Praeger Publishers, 1980), pp. 69-93.

9. See Ross D. Parke & Douglas B. Sawin, "Perspectives on Father-Infant Interaction," in *Handbook of Infancy*, ed. Joy Osofsky (New York: Wiley, 1978), pp. 64-68.

10. Jack Lee Rosenberg, Marjorie L. Rand & Diane Asay, Body, Self, and Soul: Sustaining Integration (Atlanta: Humanics Limited, 1985), p. 20.

CHAPTER 7

1. Maud Lindblå, "Sexlivet När Man Väntar Barn," *Vi Föräldrar*, no. 7, 1991, pp. 66-67.

2. Read more about lovemaking during pregnancy in Arlene Eisenberg, Heidi Eisenberg Murkoff & Sandee Eisenberg Hathaway, *What to Expect When You Are Expecting* (New York: Workman, 1984).

3. Maureen Murdoch *The Heroine's Journey* (Boston: Shambhala, 1990), p. 113.

4. Ibid., p. 115.

5. Adrianne Rich, *Of Woman Born* (New York: W.W. Norton, 1986), p. 34.

6. See Chapter 4.

7. Jack Lee Rosenberg, Marjorie Rand, & Diane Asay, *Body, Self, and Soul* (Atlanta: Humanics Limited, 1985), p. 233.

CHAPTER 8

1. Nancy R. Gibbs, "Bringing Up Father," *Time*, June 28, 1993, pp. 52-61.

2. Norma Radin, "Father Absence" (research review), ed. Michael E. Lamb, *The Role of the Father in Child Development*, second edition, (New York: John Wiley & Sons, 1981), pp. 409-419.

3. See, for example, Libby Lee & Arthur Colman, *Pregnancy: The Psychological Experience*, and Jerrold Lee Shapiro, *The Measure of a Man* (New York: Delacorte; 1993).

4. In Anne Pedersen & Peggy O'Mara, eds., *Being a Father: Family, Work, and Self* (Santa Fe: John Muir, 1990), pp. 3-9.

5. Shapiro, *The Measure of a Man*, p. 65.

6. It is estimated that almost 50 percent of all expectant fathers experience physical symptoms such as weight gain and back pain during their wife's pregnancy.

7. See Shapiro, *The Measure of a Man*, chapter 1.

8. See Ross D. Parke & Barbara R. Tinsley, "The Father's Role in Infancy: Determinants of Involvement in Caregiving and Play," in Lamb, *The Role of the Father in Child Development*, pp. 429-457.

9. Martin Greenberg, *The Birth of a Father* (New York: Continuum, 1985), p. 19.

10. Sam Keen, *Fire in the Belly: On Being a Man* (New York: Bantam Books, 1991), p. 219.

11. In Charles Scull, ed., *Fathers, Sons, and Daughters* (Los Angeles: Jeremy P. Tarcher, 1992), pp. 26-27.

12. Robert Bly, *Iron John* (New York: Vintage Books, 1990), p. 2.

13. Keen, Fire in the Belly, p. 214.

14. Shapiro, *The Measure of a Man*, p. 10.

15. Bly, *Iron John*, p. 6.

16. Clarissa Pinkola Estes, *Women Who Run with the Wolves* (New York: Ballantine, 1992), p. 7.

17. In Scull, ed., *Fathers, Sons, and Daughters*, p. 28.

18. Linda Leonard, *The Wounded Woman: Healing the FatherDaughter Relationship* (Boston: Shambhala, 1985), pp. 81-82.

19. Scull, *Fathers, Sons, and Daughters*, p. 208.

20. *Father hunger* is a term commonly used in men's studies to describe men's yearning for a meaningful connection to their fathers.

CHAPTER 9

1. Jane Price, *Motherhood: What It Does to Your Mind* (London: Pandora, 1988), p. 23.

2. Jane Swigart, *The Myth of the Bad Mother: The Emotional Realities of Mothering* (New York: Doubleday, 1991), p. 14.

3. On the origin of human consciousness, see Erich Neumann, *The Great Mother* (Princeton, N. J., Princeton University Press, 1991).

4. Carol Wallas LaChance, *The Way of the Mother* (Rockport, Mass., Element, 1991), p. 34.

5. Kathie Carlson, *In Her Image* (Boston: Shambhala, 1990), p. 21.

6. Linda Leonard, *Witness to the Fire: Creativity and the Veil of Addiction* (Boston: Shambhala, 1989), p. 335.

7. Sue Bender, *Plain and Simple* (San Francisco: HarperCollins, 1989), is a wonderful little book about the plain and simple power the author found reflected in the Amish values of simplicity, humility, and clarity.

8. Quote from *The New Yorker* on the backcover of Lennart Nilsson, *A Child Is Born* (New York: Delacorte Press/Seymour Lawrence, 1990).

9. Erich Fromm, *The Art of Loving* (New York: Harper & Row, 1956), pp. 26-29.

SELECTED BIBLIOGRAPHY

Bassoff, Evelyn. *Mothering Ourselves: Help and Healing for Adult Daughters*. New York: Dutton, 1991.

de Beauvoir, Simone. *The Second Sex*. New York: Random House, 1974.

Bergum, Vangie. *Woman to Mother: A Transformation*. Granby, Massachusetts: Bergin & Garvey, 1989.

Bernard, Jesse. *The Future of Motherhood*. New York: Penguin Books, 1974.

Birkhauser-Oeri, Sibylle. *The Mother: Archetypal Image in Fairy Tales*. Toronto: Inner City Books, 1988.

Boadella, David. *Lifestreams*. New York: Routledge & Kegan Paul, 1987.

Bolen, Jean Shinoda. *Goddesses in Every Woman: A New Psychology of Women*. New York: Harper & Row, 1984.

Cassidy-Brinn, Hornstein F, & Downer, Carol. *WomanCentered Pregnancy and Birth*. Pittsburgh and San Francisco: Cleis Press, 1984.

Chernin, Kim. *The Hungry Self: Women, Eating, and Identity*. New York: Harper & Row, 1986.

Chodorow, N. *The Reproduction of Mothering: Psychoanalysis and the Sociology of Gender*. Berkeley: University of California Press, 1978.

Colman, Libby Lee & Colman, Arthur. *Pregnancy: The Psychological Experience*. New York: The Noonday Press, Farrar, Straus & Giroux, 1991.

Dinnerstein, Dorothy. *The Mermaid and the Minotaur*. New York: Harper & Row, 1986.

Dychtwald, Ken. *Bodymind*. Los Angeles: Jeremy P. Tarcher, 1986.

von Franz, Marie-Louise. *The Feminine in Fairytales*. Dallas: Spring Publications, 1972.

Friedan, Betty. *The Feminine Mystique*. New York: Dell, 1984.

Genevie, Louis E. & Genevie, Margolies E. *The Motherhood Report: How Women Feel About Being Mothers*. New York: Macmillan, 1987.

Gerson, Kathleen. *Hard Choices: How Women Decide About Work, Career and Motherhood*. Berkeley: University of California Press, 1985.

Gilligan, Carol. *In a Different Voice: Psychological Theory and Women's Development*. Cambridge, Mass.: Harvard University Press, 1982.

Horney, Karen. *Feminine Psychology*. New York: W.W. Norton, 1967.

Keleman, Stanley. *Your Body Speaks Its Mind*. New York: Simon & Schuster, 1975.

Kitzinger, Sheila. *The Experience of Childbirth*. London: Penguin, 1962.

Klaus, Marshall H., & John H. Kennel. *Maternal Infant Bonding*. Saint Louis: Mosby, 1976.

Kohut, Heinz. *The Analysis of the Self*. New York: International University Press, 1971.

Lazarre, Jane. *The Mother Knot*. Boston: Beacon Press, 1986.

Leach, Penelope. *The First Six Months*. London: Fontana Paperbacks, 1986.

Marshall, Connie C. *From Here to Maternity*. New York: Prima/ Random House, 1991.

Matthews, Sanford J., & Bucknum Brinley, MaryAnn. *Through the Motherhood Maze*. New York: Doubleday, 1982.

Miller, Alice. *The Drama of the Gifted Child*. New York: Basic Books, 1981.

Nilsson, Lennart. *A Child Is Born*. New York: Delacorte Press/Seymour Lawrence, 1990.

Queenan, John T, ed. *A New Life: Pregnancy, Birth, and Your Child's First Year*. Boston: Little, Brown, 1986.

Rabuzzi, Kathryn Allen. *Motherself: A Mythic Analysis of Motherhood*. Bloomington: Indiana University Press, 1988.

Rothman, Barbara Katz. *Recreating Motherhood: Ideology and Technology in a Patri-archial Society*, 1989.

Rubin, Nancy. *The Mother Mirror: How a Generation of Women Is Changing Motherhood in America*. New York: Putnam, 1984.

Ruddick, Sara. *Maternal Thinking*. New York: Ballantine Books, 1989.

Satir, Virginia. *Peoplemaking*. Palo Alto, Calif.: Science and Behavior Books, 1972.

Ulanov, Ann Beford. *The Feminine in Jungian Psychology and in Christian Theology*. Evanston, Ill.: Northwestern University Press, 1971.

Weston, Carol. *From Here to Maternity: Confessions of a First Time Mother*. Boston: Little, Brown, 1991.

Winnicott, Donald W. *Collected Papers*. New York: Basic Books, 1956.

Worth, Cecilia. *The Birth of a Father: New Fathers Talk About Pregnancy, Childbirth and the First Three Months*. New York: McGraw-Hill, 1988.

INDEX

About the Author

MERETE LEONHARDT-LUPA is a psychotherapist in private practice in the Boulder, Colorado area. She specializes in parenting issues. She has a special interest in depth (Jungian) therapy with symbolic orientation and centers her work on the body and the concept of womanhood. She is the mother of three children.